IMMUNOLOGY
AN ILLUSTRATED OUTLINE
THIRD EDITION
DAVID MALE MA PhD

Senior Lecturer in Neuroimmunology
Department of Neuropathology
Institute of Psychiatry
London, UK

Publisher	Dianne Zack
Development Editor	Louise Crowe
Project Managers	Linda Horrell, Tuan Ho
Designer	Paul Phillips
Layout Artist	Lara Last
Cover Design	Greg Smith
Cover Illustration	Danny Pyne
Illustration	Lynda Payne
Production	Gudrun Hughes
Index	Anita Reid

ISBN 0 7234 2617 1

Third Edition Copyright © Mosby, an imprint of Mosby International (a division of Times Mirror International Publishers Ltd), 1998.

First published in 1986 by Gower Medical Publishing Ltd; ISBN 0 906923 58 1; reprinted 1987.

Second Edition published in 1991 by Gower Medical Publishing Ltd; ISBN 0 397 44825 2; reprinted 1993 by Mosby–Year Book Europe Ltd; reprinted 1994 by Mosby, an imprint of Times Mirror International Publisers Ltd.

Third Edition published in 1998 by Mosby, an imprint of Mosby International (a division of Times Mirror International Publishers Ltd), Lynton House, 7–12 Tavistock Square, London WC1H 9LB, UK.

Printed in Italy by Vincenzo Bona, 1998.
Text and captions set in Univers, 9pt.

Cataloguing in Publication Data
Catalogue records for this book are available from the British Library and the US Library of Congress.

How to Use this Book

This book serves two different functions. It can be used either as a dictionary of immunology or as a concise revision guide/study aid. Readers who already know some immunology and require a summary of particular aspects should consult the contents pages. The book is divided into five chapters, each of which contains a number of related topics.

To use the book as a dictionary, look up the word or abbreviation in the Index of Terms (pages vii to xiv). This gives a single page number where a definition of the word will be found – associated words will be found on the same page. Italicized numbers refer to entries within tabular figures. Page references to particular topics set out on several pages are indicated in bold.

Acknowledgements

I am most grateful to my coeditors Professor Ivan Roitt and Dr Jonathan Brostoff for letting me use or adapt some of the illustrations which appear in our book *Immunology, Fifth Edition*. I would like to thank the contributors who inspired those diagrams, including Professors Marc Feldmann, Frank Hay, Peter Lydyard, Graham Rook, Michael Steward and Malcolm Turner, and Drs Anne Cooke, Michael Owen and James Howard. In addition, I would like to thank Dr B. Greenwood, Professor C.H.W. Horne, Dr B. Dean, Professor L. Brent, Dr C. Hawkins, Dr Janice Taverne, Dr D.R. Davis, Dr R.J. Poljak, Dr D. McClaren and Mr P. Penfold for original micrographs and illustrations of pathology.

Naturally, a book of this kind cannot include everything of interest to immunologists; I have tried to cover all the essential areas of the subject, but I should be pleased to know when readers consider that particular subjects deserve further detail.

Contents

4. Immunopathology

5. Immunological Techniques

Index of Terms

NB **Bold** numbers identify sections; roman numbers identify definitions; *italic* numbers identify entries in figures or tables.

IMMUNOLOGY
An Illustrated
Outline

The Immune System | 1

INTRODUCTION

The function of the immune system is to protect the body from damage caused by microorganisms – bacteria, viruses, fungi and parasites. This defensive function is performed by leucocytes (white blood cells) and a number of accessory cells, which are distributed throughout the body, but are found particularly in lymphoid organs, including the bone marrow, thymus, spleen, lymph nodes and mucosa-associated lymphoid tissues (MALT). Lymphoid organs are strategically placed to protect different areas of the body from infection. Cells migrate between these tissues via the blood stream and lymphatic system. As they do so, they interact with each other to generate coordinated immune responses aimed at eliminating pathogens or minimizing the damage they cause.

Lymphocytes are the key cells controlling the immune response. They specifically recognize 'foreign' material and distinguish it from the body's own components. Generally they react to foreign material but not against the body's tissue. Lymphocytes are of two main types: B cells which produce antibodies, and T cells which have a number of functions including: 1) Helping B cells to make antibody; 2) Recognizing and destroying cells infected with viruses; 3) Activating phagocytes to destroy pathogens they have taken up; and 4) Controlling the level and quality of the immune response. Lymphocytes recognize foreign material by specific cell-surface antigen receptor molecules. To recognize specifically the enormous variety of different molecules, the antigen receptors must be equally diverse. Each lymphocyte makes only one type of antigen receptor, and thus can only recognize a very limited number of antigens, but as the receptors differ on each clone of cells, the lymphocyte population as a whole has an enormous number of different, specific antigen receptors.

Phagocytes include blood monocytes, macrophages and neutrophils. Their function is to take up pathogens, antigens and cell debris and to break them down. Antibodies and complement components bound to particles facilitate this process, and macrophages can also present internalized antigens to T lymphocytes.

Accessory cells include eosinophil and basophil granulocytes, mast cells, platelets and antigen-presenting cells (APCs). Eosinophils have a role in damaging some parasites and controlling inflammation. Basophils, mast cells and platelets contain a variety of molecules that mediate inflammation, and so are important in linking immune responses to inflammatory reactions. APCs include several cell types which present antigen to lymphocytes. All these cell types interact to generate an effective immune response.

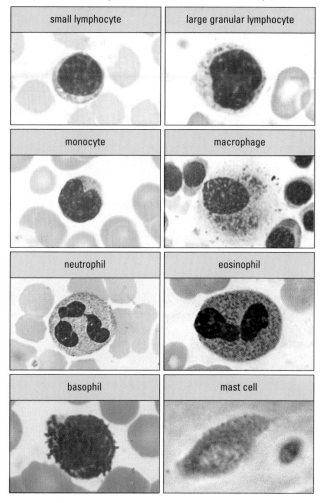

Fig. 1.1 Cells involved in the immune response. Macrophage courtesy of Professor A. V. Hoffbrand.

LYMPHOCYTES

B cells are lymphocytes which develop in foetal liver and subsequently in bone marrow. In birds, B cells develop in a specialized organ, the bursa of Fabricius. Mature B cells carry surface immunoglobulin which acts as their antigen receptor. They are distributed throughout the secondary lymphoid tissues, particularly in the follicles of lymph nodes and spleen. They respond to antigenic stimuli by dividing and differentiating into plasma cells.

Plasma cells/Antibody-Forming Cells (AFCs) are terminally differentiated B cells. They have an expanded cytoplasm with characteristic parallel arrays of rough endoplasmic reticulum and are entirely devoted to the production of secreted antibody. Plasma cells are seen in the red pulp of the spleen, the medulla of lymph nodes, the MALT and occasionally in sites of inflammation.

B-1 and B-2 cells are B cell subsets. In man, the majority of B cells are derived from bone marrow stem cells, but a minor population (B-1), distinguished by the CD5 marker, appear to form a self-renewing set. B-1 cells develop early, respond to a number of common microbial antigens and sometimes generate autoantibodies. In mice, B-1 cells respond to a particular group of T-independent antigens. In adults, the majority of B cells are of the B-2 subset. They generate a greater diversity of antigen receptors and respond well to T-dependent antigens.

T cells are lymphocytes which develop in the thymus. This organ is seeded by lymphocytic stem cells from the bone marrow during embryonic development. These cells then develop their T cell antigen receptors (TCRs) and differentiate into the two major peripheral T cell subsets, one of which expresses the CD4 marker and the other CD8. T cells can also be differentiated into two populations depending on whether they use an $\alpha\beta$ (TCR2) or a $\gamma\delta$ (TCR1) antigen receptor. The essential role of T cells is to recognize antigens originating from within cells of the host.

$\gamma\delta$ **T cells** express the $\gamma\delta$ form of the TCR. They form a minor population (<5%) of the total T cells, but constitute a greater proportion in particular sites, including the gut, skin and vagina. They appear to branch early from the main thymic developmental pathway. $\gamma\delta$ T cells appear to recognize different antigens than $\alpha\beta$ T cells, including carbohydrate and intact protein antigens. Some $\gamma\delta$ T cells do not require antigen to be processed or to be presented by major histocompatibility complex (MHC) molecules.

T cytotoxic (Tc) cells are capable of destroying virally infected target cells, or allogeneic cells. The majority of Tc cells are CD8[+] and recognize antigen on the target cell surface associated with MHC class I molecules.

T helper (TH) cells. These T lymphocytes help B cells to divide, differentiate and produce antibody. They also release cytokines which control the development of leucocyte lines from haemopoietic stem cells. Other cytokines are required for the development of cytotoxic T cells and cause activation of macrophages, allowing them to destroy the pathogens they have taken up. The majority of TH cells are CD4[+] and recognize antigen presented on the surface of APCs in association with class II molecules encoded by the MHC.

TH0/TH1/TH2 cells are subsets of TH cells differentiated *in vitro* according to the blends of cytokines they produce. TH1 cells interact most effectively with mononuclear phagocytes, while TH2 cells release cytokines which are particularly required for B cell differentiation. Both types can promote development of cytotoxic cells. TH1 and TH2 cells are thought to develop from TH0 cells, which produce a more limited profile of cytokines.

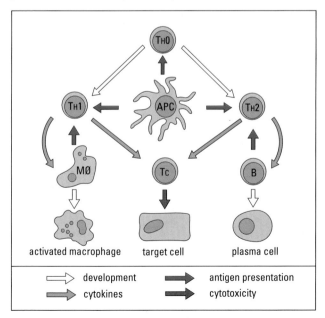

Fig. 1.2 Lymphocyte interactions.

Clonal selection describes the way in which particular lymphocytes are activated. During development, each lymphocyte generates an antigen receptor with a single antigen specificity, but the entire population of cells has a very wide range of specificities. An antigen binds specifically to only a few cells. These clones alone are stimulated to divide, so providing a large pool of effector cells and memory cells. Thus antigen selects specific clones that react against it.

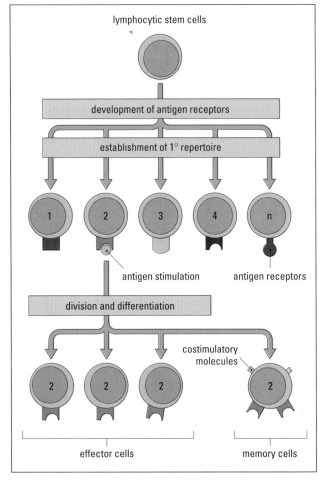

Fig. 1.3 Clonal selection and lymphocyte development.

Naive/Virgin lymphocytes are cells which have not encountered their specific antigen. They express high molecular weight variants of leucocyte common antigen (eg. CD45RA).

Memory cells are populations of long-lived T cells or B cells which have been previously stimulated by antigen and which make an accelerated response to that antigen if they encounter it again. Memory B cells carry surface IgG as their antigen receptor, and this is of higher affinity than the IgD and IgM on virgin lymphocytes. Memory T cells express the CD45RO variant of the leucocyte common antigen, as well as increased levels of adhesion molecules, including LFA-3 and VLA-4.

T suppressor (Ts) cells are functionally defined T cells which downregulate the actions of other T cells and B cells. There is no unique marker for this group of cells, and it is thought that suppression may be a facet of the actions of T_H and T_C cells.

Null (non-T, non-B) cells/L cells/Third population cells are all descriptions of a distinct population of leucocytes constituting 14% of blood mononuclear cells. They lack conventional antigen receptors, but express some markers from both the T cell and mononuclear phagocyte lineages. Nevertheless, they are thought to constitute a distinct lineage. These cells have a high density of Fc receptors (FcγRIII), which permits them to recognize and kill target cells coated with antibody. Seventy to eighty per cent of these cells have the appearance of large granular lymphocytes.

Large Granular Lymphocytes (LGLs) are morphologically defined lymphocytes, containing large amounts of cytoplasm with azurophilic granules. They constitute 5–15% of blood mononuclear cells, and correspond largely with mature null cells. This population has particular K cell and NK cell activity.

K (Killer) cells are mononuclear cells that can kill target cells sensitized with antibody, which they engage via their Fc receptors. The majority are null cells, although macrophages or eosinophils can also have K cell activity.

NK (Natural Killer) cells are capable of killing a variety of virally infected and transformed target cells to which they have not been previously sensitized. They recognize targets using several receptors, including CD2, CD69 and NKR-P1, as well as the Fc receptor CD16 (see K cells). They also receive inhibitory signals from MHC class I on potential target cells, transduced via killer inhibitory receptor (KIR; human) or Ly-49 (mouse) on the NK cell.

MARKERS

CD system. Leucocytes are differentiated by their cell surface molecules identified by monoclonal antibodies. The most readily accessible marker of lymphocytes is their antigen receptor – B cells use surface immunoglobulin, and T cells carry the T cell antigen receptor (TCR). Most other markers are designated according to the CD system of nomenclature. Some of these markers are specific for individual populations of cells, or particular phases of cellular differentiation. Others appear only on activated or dividing cells. Many of the CD markers are present at varying levels on several different cell types, so that each subset of lymphocytes expresses a unique overall profile of surface markers.

More than 200 individual molecules are recognized in the CD series, and some of them are found on cells other than leucocytes. The tables below and opposite give the identity and cellular distribution of the more important CD molecules. Particularly important are the molecules used to distinguish T cells (CD2, CD3), the principal T cell subsets (CD4, CD8), activated T cells (CD25), B cells (CD19, CD20) and mononuclear phagocytes (CD64, CD68).

Ly system defines some antigens recognized on B cells (Lyb) or T cells (Lyt) of mice. Some, but not all, correspond to CD markers.

	identity/function	T cell	B cell	NK cell	monocyte/macrophage	granulocyte	others
CD2	binds CD58 or CD48; costimulation	▢					
CD3	TCR; signal transduction	▢					
CD4	MHC class II receptor	◹					
CD5	differentiates B cell subset						
CD8	MHC class I receptor	◹					
CD11a	LFA-1; integrin α chain						
CD11b	CR3 (Mac-1); integrin α chain						
CD11c	CR4; integrin α chain						
CD15	Lewis X/sialyl LeX; binds E-selectin						
CD16	FcγRIII			▢			
CD18	β₂ integrin (see CD11)						
CD19	B cell coreceptor complex (see CD21 & 81)		▢				
CD20	B cell regulation		▢				
CD21	CR2; B cell coreceptor complex						FDC
CD23	FcεRII				★	Eo	
CD25	IL-2R α chain	★	★		★		
CD28	binds CD80; costimulation			★			

Fig. 1.4 CD markers.

	identity/function	T cell	B cell	NK cell	monocyte/ macrophage	granulocyte	others
CD29	β₁ integrin (see CD49)						
CD31	PECAM; regulates adhesion						End
CD32	FcγRII						
CD34	binds CD62L						End
CD35	CR1						FDC
CD40	binds CD40L; costimulation						IDC
CD40L	binds CD40	★				Eo B	
CD43	leukosialin						
CD44	matrix adhesion						
CD45	leucocyte common antigen (LCA)						
CD45R	restricted LCA						
CD46	membrane cofactor protein (MCP)						
CD48	binds CD2 (mouse)						
CD49a	VLA-1; integrin α chain	★					
CD49b	VLA-2; integrin α chain	★					
CD49c	VLA-3; integrin α chain						
CD49d	VLA-4; binds VCAM-1 & fibronectin	★					
CD49e	VLA-5; integrin binds fibronectin						
CD49f	VLA-6; integrin binds laminin						
CD50	ICAM-3; costimulation						
CD54	ICAM-1; adhesion	★	★	★			End
CD55	DAF						
CD56	NCAM; adhesion	★	★				
CD57	HNK-1						
CD58	LFA-3; costimulation						
CD59	protectin						
CD62E	E-selectin						End
CD62P	P-selectin						End
CD62L	L-selectin						
CD64	FcγRI						
CD68	macrosialin						
CD71	transferrin receptor	★	★	★	★		★
CD74	MHC class II-associated chain						IDC
CD79ab	sIg; signal transduction						
CD80	binds CD28; costimulation						
CD81	TAPA; B cell coreceptor complex						
CD89	FcαR						
CD90	Thy-1						Thy
CD95	binds CD95L; cytotoxicity						
CD102	ICAM-2						End
CD106	VCAM-1						End

Key	☐ Useful marker	◹ Subpopulation	★ Activated cells

B=Basophil   End=Endothelium   Eo=Eosinophil   FDC=Follicular dendritic cell
IDC=Interdigitating dendritic cell   Thy=Thymocytes

ANTIGEN-PRESENTING CELLS

Antigen-presenting cells (APCs) are a group of functionally defined cells which are capable of taking up antigens and presenting them to lymphocytes in a form they can recognize. Some antigens are taken up by APCs in the periphery and transported to the secondary lymphoid tissues, while other APCs are normally resident in these tissues and intercept antigen as it arrives. Whereas B cells recognize antigen in its native form, TH cells recognize antigenic peptides which have become associated with MHC molecules. Consequently, in order to present antigen to a TH cell, an APC must internalize it, process it into fragments, and re-express it at the cell surface in association with class II MHC molecules. In addition, many APCs provide costimulatory signals to lymphocytes, either by direct cellular interactions or by cytokines. Dendritic cells, macrophages, B cells and sometimes even tissue cells can present antigen to TH cells.

Dendritic Cells (DCs) are a distinct set of APCs distributed in many tissues of the body. The interdigitating dendritic cell (IDC), located in T cell areas of lymph node, is a member of this lineage. IDCs express class II MHC molecules and costimulatory molecules (eg. B7) so that they are very effective in presenting antigen to virgin CD4$^+$ T cells. It is thought that tissue dendritic cells migrate to lymph nodes, carrying antigen, and there upregulate molecules required for T cell activation.

Langerhans' cells (Veiled cells) are APCs of the skin which pick up antigen and transport it to regional lymph nodes. They express CD1 and high levels of MHC class II molecules and have a characteristic racket-shaped granule, the Birbeck granule (function unknown). In afferent lymph they are seen as veiled cells, and in lymph nodes they develop into dendritic cells. They are particularly important in the development of contact hypersensitivity, and skin-sensitizing agents induce their emigration from skin.

Macrophage APCs. Macrophages phagocytose antigens and some of them can also process and present it. MHC class II expression is induced following activation by microbial compounds. The recirculating macrophages of secondary lymphoid tissues are mostly seen in the medulla of lymph nodes and the red pulp of spleen. They are particularly effective in presenting antigens to TH1 cells which have been previously sensitized by dendritic cells. Activated macrophages upregulate costimulatory molecules, including B7 and ICAM-1, and secrete IL-1.

Follicular Dendritic Cells (FDCs) are present in spleen and lymph node follicles, where they appear tightly surrounded by lymphocytes. Complement-fixing immune complexes localize on the surface of these cells via Fc and C3 receptors, where they are presented mainly to B cells. This form of complex localization and presentation is important in the development of B cell memory.

Iccosomes are beaded cytoplasmic structures present on filopodia of FDCs, which are thought to act as a long-term repository for antigens. They bud off and may be internalized by B cells.

Marginal zone macrophages are present in the marginal zone of the splenic periarteriolar lymphatic sheath and along the marginal sinus of lymph nodes. T-independent antigens such as polysaccharides tend to localize on these cells, where they are often very persistent. They present antigens primarily to B cells.

Facultative APCs. Many cells of the body can be induced to express MHC class II when stimulated by IFN-γ. Sometimes they can present antigen to CD4$^+$ T cells, although they often fail to induce T cell division, due to their inability to deliver costimulatory signals. Antigen presentation by such cells may make them susceptible to cytotoxicity by the T cells.

APC	location	MHC class II	costimulatory molecules	present to:
interdigitating dendritic cell	lymph node paracortex	++	B7.1 B7.2 ICAM-1 ICAM-3	naive T cell
B cell	germinal centre	+ →++	B7.1 B7.2 ICAM-1 inducible	T cell
macrophage	tissues and lymphoid organs	0 →++	B7 inducible ICAM-3 ICAM-1 inducible	T cell
marginal zone macrophage	marginal zone of spleen and lymph node	–	–	T-ind ags →B cell
follicular dendritic cell	germinal centre	–	iccosome components (eg. C3b)	B cell

Fig. 1.5 Antigen-presenting cells.

PHAGOCYTES AND AUXILIARY CELLS

Mononuclear Phagocyte System (MPS)/Reticuloendothelial system is the collective term for the long-lived phagocytic cells distributed throughout the organs of the body. They are derived from bone marrow stem cells and express receptors for immunoglobulin (FcγRI) and complement (CR1, CR3 and often CR4). They phagocytose antigenic particles and some have the ability to present antigen to lymphocytes. This group includes:

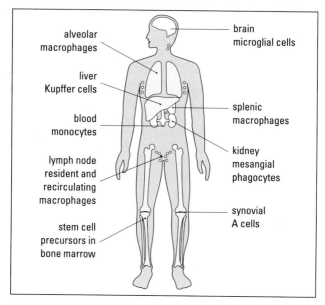

alveolar macrophages

liver Kupffer cells

blood monocytes

lymph node resident and recirculating macrophages

stem cell precursors in bone marrow

brain microglial cells

splenic macrophages

kidney mesangial phagocytes

synovial A cells

Fig. 1.6 Mononuclear phagocyte system.

Monocytes are circulating cells, constituting about 5% of total blood leucocytes, which can migrate into tissues to become macrophages. These cells have a horseshoe-shaped nucleus, azurophilic granules and many lysosomes.

Macrophages are large phagocytic cells found in most tissues and lining serous cavities and the lung. Resident macrophages may remain in tissues for years, whereas others recirculate through secondary lymphoid tissues, where they may function as APCs.

Kupffer cells are phagocytes which lie along the liver sinusoids. Much of the antigen entering the body through the gut is removed by these cells.

Mesangial phagocytes line the glomerular endothelium where the capillaries enter the Bowman's capsule.

Microglial cells are resident phagocytes of brain. Colonization occurs primarily before birth and in the neonatal period.

Synovial A cells are phagocytes which lie on the synovium, in contact with the synovial fluid.

Granulocytes (Polymorphs), recognizable by their multilobed nuclei and numerous cytoplasmic granules, constitute the majority of blood leucocytes. They are classified by staining as:

Neutrophils – professional phagocytes and the most abundant of the leucocytes (>70%). They spend less than 48 hours in the circulation before migrating into the tissues under the influence of chemotactic stimuli, where they phagocytose material and eventually die. They have receptors for antibody and complement, to facilitate the uptake of opsonized particles.

Eosinophils – comprising 2–5% of blood leucocytes. Their granules contain a crystalloid core of basic protein which can be released by exocytosis, causing damage to a number of pathogens, particularly parasites. The granules also contain histaminase and aryl sulphatase, which downregulate inflammatory reactions.

Basophils – constituting <0.5% of blood leucocytes. Their granules contain inflammatory mediators and they are in some ways functionally similar to mast cells.

Mast cells are present in most tissues adjoining the blood vessels. They contain numerous granules with inflammatory mediators such as histamine and PAF, released by triggering with C3a and C5a, or by crosslinking of surface IgE bound to their high-affinity IgE receptor (FcεRI). Stimulation also causes them to produce prostaglandins and leukotrienes. There are two types of mast cell, thought to be derived from a common precursor:

Connective Tissue Mast Cells (CTMCs) – the main tissue-fixed mast cell population. They are ubiquitous, distributed around blood vessels and contain large amounts of histamine and heparin. They are inhibitable by sodium cromoglycate.

Mucosal Mast Cells (MMCs) – present in the gut and lung. They are dependent on IL-3 and IL-4 for their proliferation and are increased during parasitic infections.

LYMPHOID SYSTEM

Primary and Secondary lymphoid tissue. Lymphocytes are derived from bone marrow stem cells, and initially develop in the primary lymphoid tissues – T cells in the thymus and B cells in bone marrow. Mature cells expressing antigen receptors seed the secondary lymphoid tissues, the spleen, lymph nodes and collections of mucosa-associated lymphoid tissues (MALT).

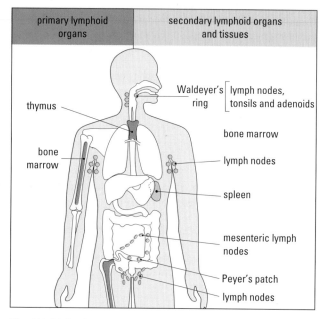

Fig. 1.7 Major lymphoid organs and tissues.

Lymphocyte traffic. Lymphocytes leave the circulation by traversing specialized venules (HEVs) in the lymph nodes and MALT. They recirculate via the lymphatic system, through chains of lymph nodes, back to the circulation. Recirculation gives lymphocytes the opportunity to contact their antigen.

High Endothelial Venules (HEVs) are present in most secondary lymphoid tissues, and may be induced in other tissues during severe, persistent immune reactions. They are lined by distinctive columnar cells, expressing site-specific sets of glycosylated adhesion molecules (eg. glyCAM-1, MAdCAM-1). Up to 25% of lymphocytes passing through secondary lymphoid tissues bind to these molecules and migrate across HEVs.

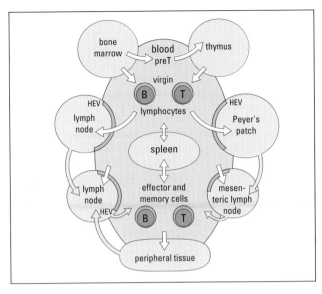

Fig. 1.8 Lymphocyte traffic.

Lymphatic system is the system of vessels covering the entire body, which is responsible for draining tissues and returning the transudate to the blood. It also acts as a route for the movement of antigens from the periphery to lymph nodes, and for the recirculation of lymphocytes and dendritic cells.

Thoracic duct and Right lymphatic duct are the main lymphatic vessels draining into the blood. Recirculating cells from the trunk, internal organs and lower limbs pass through the thoracic duct into the left subclavian vein. The right lymphatic duct drains the upper right segment of the body.

Mucosa-Associated Lymphoid Tissue (MALT) is a general term for the unencapsulated lymphoid tissues that are seen in submucosal areas of the respiratory, gastrointestinal and urinogenitary systems. These protect potential sites of pathogen invasion.

Waldeyer's ring is the term for the lymphoid tissue of the neck and pharynx, which includes the adenoids, tonsils and regional lymph nodes.

Tonsils and Adenoids are pharyngeal parts of the MALT that are particularly rich in B cells arranged into lymphoid follicles.

LEUCOCYTE DEVELOPMENT

Bone marrow is a haemopoietic tissue present in long bones and the axial skeleton. A network of venous sinuses is arranged around a central artery and vein and these permeate the developing cells. All blood cells are derived from bone marrow stem cells, and 10% of the marrow cells are lymphocytes, occurring in clusters around the radial arteries. In adult mammals, B cells develop and differentiate in the marrow. Stromal cells secrete cytokines required for leucocyte development, including stem cell factor (SCF) and IL-7 required for the early development of pre-T and pre-B cells. Small numbers of mature lymphocytes also reside in the marrow.

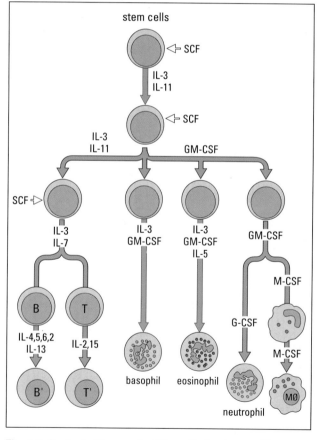

Fig. 1.9 Control of leucocyte differentiation by cytokines.

Stem Cell Factor (SCF, Steel factor) is a cytokine which acts on a variety of lineages to promote division. Differentiating cells lose their requirement for SCF.

c-Kit (CD117) is the receptor for SCF, present on T cell and B cell precursors, which has an intracytoplasmic tyrosine kinase domain. It disappears when the lymphocyte precursors start to recombine their antigen receptor genes. A subpopulation of NK cells expresses c-Kit permanently. Mast cell precursors also express c-Kit, which also binds mast cell growth factor (MGF).

Colony-Stimulating Factors (CSFs) control the differentiation of haemopoietic stem cells, both in the bone marrow and in the periphery (see opposite). This group of cytokines includes granulocyte, macrophage and granulocyte/macrophage CSFs (G-CSF, M-CSF and GM-CSF, respectively), which promote the differentiation of their specific subsets of leucocytes. In addition, IL-3 (pan-specific haemopoietin), IL-5, IL-7, IL-11 and erythropoietin are functional members of this group.

Myeloid cells are the granulocyte and mononuclear phagocyte lineages which develop from a common stem cell. The stem cell (CFU-GM) expresses CD34 (also present on resting endothelium) and MHC class II, which is lost as differentiation proceeds.

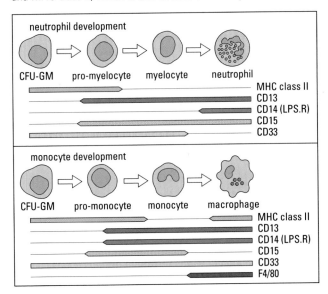

Fig. 1.10 Differentiation of myeloid cells.

THYMUS

The thymus is a primary lymphoid organ overlying the heart, seeded by lymphoid stem cells from the bone marrow, which differentiate into T cells. It is bilobed and organized into lobules separated by connective tissue septae (trabeculae). Each lobule is divided into cortex and medulla.

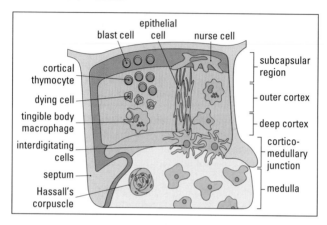

Fig. 1.11 The structure of a thymus lobule.

Thymocytes are thymic lymphocytes. The repertoire of T cell antigen receptors develops and the deletion of autoreactive cells occurs, during T cell maturation in the thymus, by interaction with APCs. The process involves proliferation of immature cells, but many cells die (by apoptosis) during selection.

Thymic cortex. The outer zone of the thymus contains about 85% of the total thymocytes. The cells are immature, express CD1 in man and divide rapidly.

Thymic medulla contains relatively few lymphocytes, but they are more mature than those in the cortex, and the peripheral T cell populations (CD4$^+$ or CD8$^+$) start to emerge here.

Thymic epithelial cells are a network of MHC class II-bearing APCs extending throughout the cortex and medulla, which are involved in the selection of the T cell repertoire.

Hassall's corpuscles are whorled structures, possibly of epithelial cells, seen in the medulla. Their function is unknown.

T CELL DEVELOPMENT

Education of T cells occurs in the thymus. Pre-T cells seed the thymus from the bone marrow and proliferate in the subcapsular region. These cells are CD4$^-$,8$^-$ but they develop into the rapidly proliferating CD4$^+$,8$^+$ (double positive) cortical population, which constitutes the majority of thymocytes. They generate their antigen receptors (TCRs), and undergo positive and negative selection. The differentiating thymocytes lose either CD4 or CD8, leaving mature T cells expressing CD4 or CD8 only (single positive), seen in the medulla. Cells which fail to generate a functional TCR or which cannot interact with self MHC, or which recognize self antigens, die during development in the cortex, to be phagocytosed by tingible body macrophages.

Positive and Negative selection are the processes by which thymocytes are rescued from apoptosis during development. Cells are positively selected by interaction with MHC molecules on thymic epithelial cells and negatively selected if they recognize a self antigen presented by MHC molecules on dendritic cells acting as APCs.

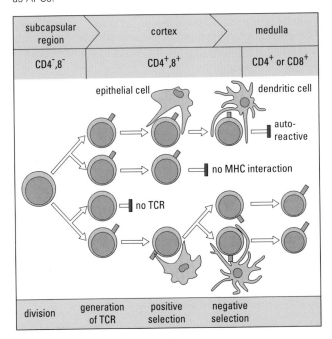

Fig. 1.12 T cell development in the thymus.

LYMPH NODES

Lymph nodes are encapsulated organs which punctuate the lymphoid network and contain aggregations of lymphocytes and APCs. They are strategically placed to intercept antigens from the periphery and there are large groups of lymph nodes in the axillae, groin and neck. The mesenteric lymph nodes are very large, and well sited to protect the body from antigen and pathogens from the gut. Lymph nodes are structurally organized into different areas:

Marginal sinus lies immediately beneath the capsule and is lined by phagocytic cells, the marginal zone macrophages, which can trap antigens entering the node.

Cortex, the outer region of the lymph node, contains mainly B cells. Follicles lie within this region.

Paracortex contains mainly T cells, interspersed with interdigitating cells expressing high levels of MHC class II antigens, which present antigen to the T cells.

Medulla contains relatively fewer lymphocytes and more macrophages and plasma cells than other regions. Medullary cords are strands of lymphocytes, both B cells and T cells, which extend into the medulla.

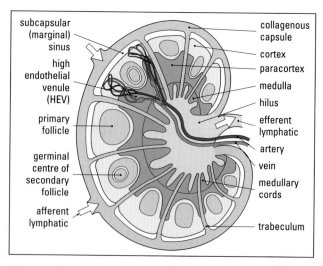

Fig. 1.13 The structure of a lymph node.

Afferent and Efferent lymphatics. Cells arrive in the lymph nodes via HEVs and afferent lymphatics which drain into the marginal (subcapsular) sinus. They migrate into specialized areas and finally leave by the efferent lymphatic vessel.

Lymphoid follicles are aggregations of closely packed lymphocytes and APCs. Unstimulated lymph nodes contain primary follicles, which develop into expanded secondary follicles after antigen stimulation.

Germinal centres are regions of rapidly proliferating cells seen in the centre of secondary follicles, and are important in the development of B cell memory and the secondary antibody response. A few B cells initiate the germinal centre. They undergo rapid division in the basal dark zone (centroblasts). This is associated with somatic mutation of the immunoglobulin genes. The diversified cells become centrocytes in the basal light zone where they may take up antigen released from follicular dendritic cells. B cells with high-affinity antibody are selected, while those with low-affinity antibody die and are phagocytosed by macrophages. Centrocytes present antigen to the small numbers of CD4$^+$ T cells present in the germinal centre, and undergo a second phase of division before leaving via the mantle zone, to become memory cells or plasma cells.

Bcl-2 is a molecule induced on centrocytes which have taken up antigen. Ligation of Bcl-2 rescues the cell from apoptosis. Bcl-2 is also expressed on developing haemopoietic cells in marrow.

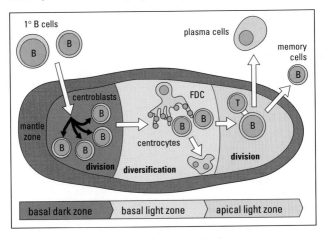

Fig. 1.14 B cell development in a germinal centre.

SPLEEN

The spleen is an encapsulated secondary lymphoid organ which lies in the peritoneum, beneath the diaphragm and behind the stomach. It contains two types of tissue, termed the red pulp and the white pulp or periarteriolar lymphatic sheath (PALS).

Red pulp consists of a network of splenic cords and venous sinuses lined by macrophages, which effect the destruction of effete erythrocytes. Plasma cells may also be seen in this region.

White pulp/PALS (Periarteriolar Lymphatic Sheath) contains the majority of the lymphoid tissue, distributed around the arterioles. T cells are found mainly around the central arterioles, and B cells are further out. The B cells may be organized into primary and secondary lymphoid follicles, with germinal centres. Phagocytes and APCs are also present in the follicles.

Marginal zone is the outer region of the PALS. It contains slowly recirculating B cells and marginal zone macrophages which present T-independent antigens to B cells. Marginal sinuses lie at the edge of the marginal zone. Most lymphocytes enter the PALS via specialized capillaries in the marginal zone and migrate out via bridging channels, between the marginal sinuses, into the venous sinuses of the red pulp.

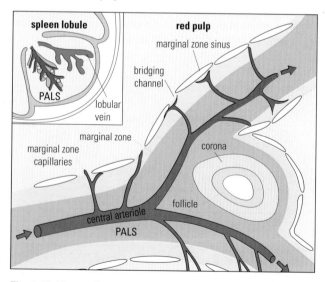

Fig. 1.15 The periarteriolar lymphatic sheath (PALS).

GALT (GUT-ASSOCIATED LYMPHOID TISSUES)

The GALT comprises the mucosa-associated lymphoid tissues of the gut. These include the focal accumulations of lymphocytes in the lamina propria and Peyer's patches, which contain disproportionately high numbers of IgA-producing B cells and plasma cells.

Peyer's patches are collections of lymphocytes in the wall of the small intestine, which appear macroscopically as pale patches on the gut wall. The adjoining part of the intestinal mucosa lacks goblet cells and has a specialized epithelium that includes a unique cell type, the M cell, which transports antigens to the underlying lymphocytes. Lymphocytes enter a patch via the HEV, which selectively expresses an adhesion molecule, MAdCAM-1, which binds lymphocytes expressing $\alpha_4\beta_7$ integrin. Lymphocytes exit the Peyer's patch via the local lymphatics and selectively localize to the lamina propria of the gut.

Secretory immune system refers to immune defences present in secretory organs, such as salivary glands, mammary glands and GALT. Their main protection is provided by secretory IgA. Dimeric IgA binds to a poly-Ig receptor on the basal surface of epithelial cells and is transported to the gut lumen.

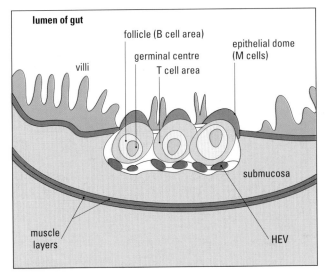

Fig. 1.16 Structure of a Peyer's patch.

Antigen Recognition | 2

ANTIGEN RECEPTORS

The immune system has two main ways of recognizing antigens. B cells recognize intact antigens using immunoglobulin (antibody) as their receptor. T cells, on the other hand, have evolved to recognize antigen originating from within other cells, using their T cell antigen receptors (TCRs).

Antigen is the term used to describe any molecule that can be recognized by the immune system. In general, immunoglobulins recognize and bind to intact antigens, or large fragments of them which have retained their tertiary structure. By contrast, T cells will only recognize polypeptide fragments of antigens which have become associated with molecules encoded by the major histocompatibility complex (MHC) and which are expressed on the surface of other cells of the body.

Antigenic determinants, or epitopes, are the parts of an antigen to which an immunoglobulin binds. Antigens usually have many determinants, which may be different from each other or be repeated molecular structures. Virtually the entire surface of a protein is potentially antigenic. Figure 2.1 illustrates epitopes on lysozyme recognized by three different monoclonal antibodies.

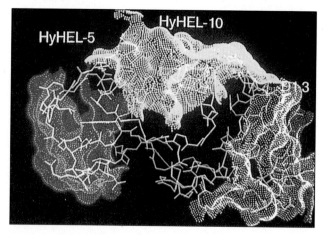

Fig. 2.1 Three epitopes of lysozyme. Courtesy of Dr D. R. Davis.

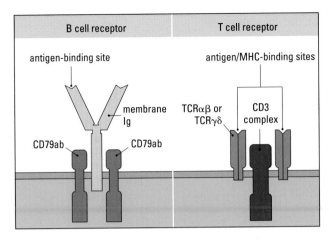

Fig. 2.2 Antigen-binding molecules.

Antibodies (Abs)/Immunoglobulins (Igs) were originally identified as a class of serum proteins induced following contact with antigen, which bind specifically to the antigen that induced their formation. Most antibodies are present in the gamma globulin fraction of serum. Subsequently, it was found that B cells use a membrane-bound form of their secreted antibody as an antigen receptor. Surface Igs on B cells are associated with two polypeptides, Igα and Igβ (CD79a and CD79b).

Igα and Igβ (CD79) are transmembrane molcules that transduce activation signals to the B cell and are required for expression of membrane Ig. Hence CD79 is a marker of mature B cells.

T cell antigen receptors (TCRs) are integral membrane proteins on all mature T cells, which specifically recognize antigenic peptides associated with MHC-encoded molecules. The receptor consists of a heterodimer responsible for antigen/MHC binding and a cluster of associated membrane-bound polypeptides called the CD3 complex that trigger cellular activation and are required for cell activation. The antigen/MHC-binding portion of the TCR varies between different clones of T cells, while the peptides of the CD3 complex are invariant.

Immunoreceptor Tyrosine-based Activation Motifs (ITAMs, ARAMs) are segments found in the intracytoplasmic sections of CD79 and CD3 which are targets for phosphorylation by tyrosine kinases, allowing them to interact with cytosolic enzymes.

ANTIBODY STRUCTURE

Heavy chains and light chains. Antibody molecules all have a basic four polypeptide chain structure, consisting of two identical light (L) chains and two identical heavy (H) chains, stabilized and crosslinked by intra-chain and inter-chain disulphide bonds (red), and the heavy chains are glycosylated (Fig. 2.3). There are five major types of Ig heavy chains (μ, γ, α, ε, δ), consisting of 450–600 amino acid residues, and the type determines the class of the antibody. Light chains are of two main types (κ, λ), consisting of about 230 residues, and either type of light chain may associate with any of the heavy chains. Both heavy and light chains are folded into domains.

Membrane and Secreted immunoglobulins. Antibodies can be produced either as integral membrane proteins of B cells, which act as their antigen receptor, or in a secreted form. Secreted Igs are structurally identical to their membrane counterparts, except that they lack the transmembrane segment and small intracytoplasmic section of amino acids at the C-terminus of membrane Ig. Secreted Igs are present in extracellular fluids and secretions. Virgin B cells produce membrane Igs, but following activation by antigen and differentiation into plasma cells, they switch to the production of secreted Igs.

Immunoglobulin supergene family. The domains in antibodies consist of three or four polypeptide loops stabilized by β-pleated

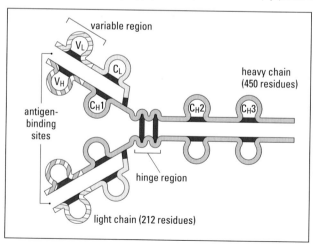

Fig. 2.3 **Polypeptide chain structure of IgG1.**

sheet and an intra-chain disulphide bond. The structure so formed is sometimes called a β-barrel. Light chains have two domains and heavy chains four or five. This structure is found in many molecules, which are said to belong to the Ig superfamily.

Hinge region is a section of the heavy chain between the Fc and Fab regions which contains the inter-heavy-chain disulphide bonds and confers segmental flexibility on the antibody molecule.

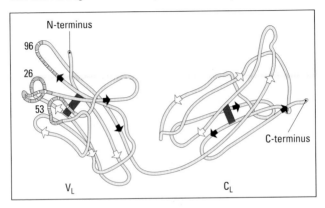

Fig. 2.4 The folding pattern of an immunoglobulin light chain.

Variable (V) and Constant (C) regions. Examination of the degree of amino acid variability between different antibody molecules of the same class shows that the largest amount of sequence variation is concentrated in the N-terminal domains of the light and heavy chains; hence this is called the V region. The V regions of one light and one heavy chain form an antigen-binding site. The remaining domains are relatively invariant within any particular class of antibody, and so are called the constant (C) region. The domains of antibody molecules are named according to whether they are in the variable or constant region of the molecules, and according to whether they are in the light or heavy chain. For example:

V_H and V_L are the variable domains of heavy and light chains.

C_L and C_H1 are the constant domains of the light chain and the first constant domain of the heavy chain, respectively.

C_γ, C_μ etc. Heavy chain domains are sometimes referred to by the class of antibody. For example $C_\mu1$ is the first constant domain of the μ heavy chain of IgM antibody.

ANTIBODY – STRUCTURAL VARIATIONS

Classes and Subclasses (Isotypes). Antibodies may be grouped on the basis of structural similarities into different classes and subclasses depending on their heavy chains. Each class sub-serves different functions. In mammals there are five antibody classes: IgG, IgM, IgA, IgD and IgE. IgG and IgA are further div-ided into subclasses. The number of subclasses varies between species. For example, in man there are four IgG subclasses, IgG1–IgG4. As there is a gene in every individual for every one of the classes and subclasses, these are isotypic variants or antibody isotypes.

Kappa and Lambda chains. Antibody light chains may also be divided into two types, namely κ and λ, which are encoded by separate gene loci. They too are isotypic variants. Either type of light chain can combine with any of the heavy chains.

Allelic exclusion is the process by which a cell uses either the gene from its maternal chromosome or the one from the paternal chromosome, but not both. Individual B cells display allelic exclusion of their heavy and light chain genes. T cells also display allelic exclusion of their TCR αβ or γδ heterodimers.

Allotypes are variants due to intraspecies genetic differences. Each individual has a particular variant at each Ig gene locus, which will often differ from those in other individuals.

Idiotypes (Ids) are variants due to the large amount of structural heterogeneity in the Ig (or TCR) V regions. This is related to the diversity required to bind different antigens. Some idiotypes are only made by animals which have particular sets of Ig genes (haplotypes) and these are called germline idiotypes.

Recurrent and Dominant idiotypes. Sometimes a particular idiotype is frequently seen in the immune response of different individuals to a particular antigen. This is a recurrent idiotype. If an idiotype constitutes a major part of an antibody response to that antigen, then it is a dominant idiotype.

Idiotopes. The V domains of antibodies can act as antigens just as any other protein, and antibodies raised against them will recog-nize antigenic determinants in their V domains. These are termed idiotopes. An idiotype is identified by the collection of idiotopes it expresses. If an idiotope is present on two different antibodies, they are said to be cross-reactive idiotypes.

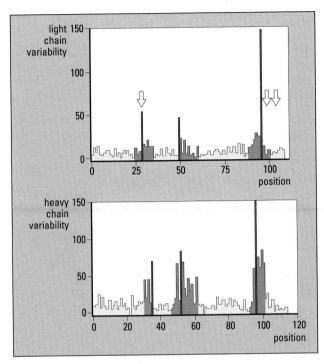

Fig. 2.5 Kabat and Wu plots of light and heavy chain variability.

Kabat and Wu plot shows the amino acid sequence variability in Igs, determined by comparing the amino acid sequences of many different antibodies. It plots variability against amino acid position, thereby highlighting the most variable regions of the heavy and light chains.

Hypervariable regions and Framework segments. The Kabat and Wu plots show that most variability is clustered in three hypervariable regions of the antibody H and L chains (red), separated by relatively invariant framework segments.

Complementarity-Determining Regions (CDRs) are the part of the V domains which form the antigen-binding site. V domain folding brings the CDRs together at the distal tip of the molecule.

Groups and Subgroups. The numerous V region domains can be classified into groups and subgroups according to similarities in the amino acid sequences of their frameworks.

ANTIBODY FUNCTIONS

Antibodies are bifunctional molecules. Their first function is to bind antigen and their second is to interact with host tissues and effector systems to facilitate removal of the antigen. Some antibody functions can be mediated just by binding to the antigen. For example, antibodies that bind to surface molecules of viruses can prevent their binding to and infecting host cells. However, most antibody functions require that the complexed antigen is bound to Fc receptors on cells. The antigen-binding sites are formed by the V domains of a heavy and light chain, whereas the C domains of the Fc region interact with cells of the immune system and C1q of the complement system. The different antibody classes and subclasses interact with different cells, and so have slightly different functions.

IgG is the major serum Ig and constitutes the main antibody in the secondary immune response to most antigens. In man, it is transferred across the placenta to provide protection in neonatal life. All IgG subclasses, except IgG4, can bind to C1q by sites in $C_\gamma 2$ to activate the complement classical pathway. IgG can act as an opsonin by crosslinking immune complexes to Fc receptors on neutrophils and macrophages. It can also sensitize target cells for destruction by K cells – large granular lymphocytes that express Fc receptors.

IgM is a pentamer of the basic four-chain structure. It is the first class to be produced during the development of the immune system and in the primary immune response. It fixes complement very efficiently and is the main antibody component of the response to T-independent antigens.

IgD is a trace antibody in serum but acts as a cell surface receptor on many B cells, where it is coexpressed with IgM. IgD appears on differentiating B cells following activation, but is absent from mature antibody-forming cells.

IgA occurs as monomers, dimers and polymers of the basic four-chain unit, existing in man mostly as monomers and in other species as dimers. IgA is the most abundant Ig class in secretions, where it protects mucous membranes. It is also found in colostrum and is particularly important in protecting the neonates of species which do not transfer IgG across the placenta.

J chain is a polypeptide present in polymeric Igs (IgM and IgA) which facilitates their polymerization. It is synthesized by B cells, but is not encoded by the Ig genes.

Poly-Ig receptor is present on the serosal surface of epithelial cells, which can transport and secrete IgA. It is a member of the Ig supergene family, which has five domains. IgA dimers bind to the receptor and are transported across the endothelium. The receptor is then cleaved, forming the secretory piece and releasing secreted IgA by exocytosis.

Secretory piece is the released form of the poly-Ig receptor, which attaches to IgA by disulphide bonds and is wound around the IgA, to protect it from degradation by enzymes.

IgE binds to high-affinity Fc receptors (FcεRI) on mast cells and basophils, where it sensitizes them to release pharmacological mediators after contact with antigen. IgE may be particularly important in protection against helminth infections, but it also mediates type I hypersensitivity reactions, such as asthma and hayfever.

immunoglobulin	heavy chain	mean serum concentration (mg/ml)	mol. wt (kDa)	number of heavy chain domains	complement C1 activation	placental transfer	epithelial transport	mast cell binding
IgG1	γ1	9	146	4	+	+		
IgG2	γ2	3	146	4	+	+		
IgG3	γ3	1	170	4	+	+		
IgG4	γ4	0.5	146	4		+		
IgM	μ	1.5	970	5	+			
IgD	δ	0.03	184	4				
IgA1	α1	3.0	160	4				
IgA2	α2	0.5	160	4				
sIgA	α1 or α2	0.05	385	4			+	
IgE	ε	0.00005	188	5				+

Fig. 2.6 Properties of human Ig isotypes.

ANTIBODY GENES

The genes for antibodies lie at three gene loci on separate chromosomes. These are the K, L (κ,λ) and H (heavy chain) loci. At each of these loci, there are large numbers of different gene segments encoding polypeptides (exons), separated by segments which do not encode protein (introns), but which contain sequences important in gene control and the process of recombination. The antibody genes undergo a number of recombinational events during B cell development and maturation. The first events are DNA rearrangements of H and L chain genes which form the gene segments encoding their V domains.

Generation of diversity refers to the process by which the large number of antibody V regions are generated. This is achieved by:
- Many different germline V genes in the K, L and H loci.
- Recombination between V, D and J gene segments.
- Insertion of non-germline (N) nucleotides into the joints.
- Varied combinations of light and heavy chains.
- Somatic mutation of V genes in individual B cells.

T cell receptors are diversified by similar mechanisms, although TCR genes are not subject to somatic mutation.

V genes encode the N-terminal 95 (approx.) amino acids of the antibody V domains. The number of V genes at each locus varies between loci and betweenspecies. Analogous V genes are present at the gene loci encoding T cell receptor (TCR) chains.

J genes and D genes. To produce a gene encoding an H-chain V domain, any one of the H-chain V-gene segments is recombined with any of a small number of D (diversity) and J (joining) genes to produce a VDJ gene. Recombination of light chains is similar, except that they have no D gene segments, and a V gene is recombined directly to a J gene. Analogous J gene segments are present in the T cell receptor A, B, G and D loci, and analogous D genes are present in the B and D loci. (Note that J gene segments should not be confused with J chains.)

Recombination and the 12/23 rule. Recombination is the process by which the various gene segments for antigen receptors are brought together and joined. This process depends on specific recombination sequences flanking each V, D and J gene, which appose the gene segments, which are enzymically cut and rejoined to remove the intervening introns. The sequences consist of a heptamer, 12 or 23 bases and a nonamer. The 12/23 rule

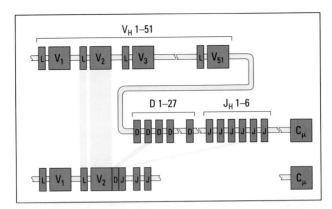

Fig. 2.7 VDJ recombination in the human *IGH* locus.

states that a flanking sequence with 12 bases can only recombine with one of 23 bases. This ensures that heavy chains only make VDJ recombinations, and light chains only VJ links.

Signal joints and Coding joints are formed during VJ or VDJ recombination. A signal joint is formed between the introns flanking the V, D or J segments, causing the intervening loop of DNA to be excised. The coding joint is formed between the recombining V, J or D exons. The precise point of the coding joint may vary, as illustrated below for the recombination of *KV21* and *KJ1* in different myelomas, giving rise to different base sequences and thus providing an additional source of diversity.

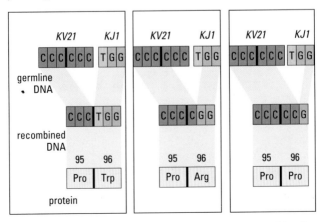

Fig. 2.8 Light chain diversity created by variable recombination.

N regions are sections of nucleotides that may be inserted into the junctions between V, D and J gene segments during recombination. They are not encoded in the germline.

RAG-1, RAG-2 (Recombination-Activating Genes) control the lineage-specific recombination of the TCR genes in T cells or the Ig genes in B cells.

Somatic hypermutation is the process by which DNA base changes occur during the lifetime of a B cell, producing point mutations in the Ig polypeptides. The high rate of mutation is centred on the recombined VJ and VDJ genes. The mechanism becomes activated in centroblasts and is associated with, but not consequent on, class switching. Thus IgG molecules usually vary more from germline sequences than IgM.

Antibody synthesis. The segment of DNA encoding the recombined VDJ (heavy chain) or VJ (light chain) region and the C region is transcribed into a primary RNA transcript, which still contains the introns. This transcript is then spliced to remove the introns, a process which involves recognition of specific base sequences called donor and acceptor junctions, immediately flanking the exons. This leaves mRNA, which is translated across the membrane of the endoplasmic reticulum (ER). Each mRNA has a leader (L) or signal sequence (SS) by which it is directed to the ER. The process is illustrated below for a membrane IgM μ polypeptide. Complete Igs are assembled and glycosylated within the ER, and stored in the Golgi apparatus. Secreted Igs are released by exocytosis, while membrane Igs associated with CD79-signalling polypeptides are moved to the cell surface.

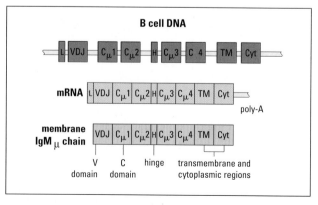

Fig. 2.9 Production of an IgM μ polypeptide.

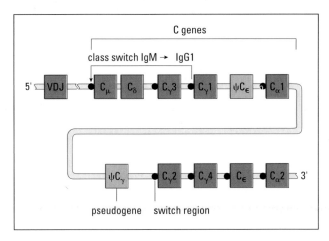

Fig. 2.10 Class switching in the human _IGH_ C gene locus.

C genes. The heavy-chain constant-region genes are arranged downstream (3′) of the recombined VDJ gene. Each gene consists of a series of exons encoding the individual C domains, as well as separate exon(s) for the hinge (except IgA) and for the transmembrane and cytoplasmic regions. The primary transcript of the heavy chains can be processed in two different ways, to produce mRNA for either membrane or secreted Ig. To produce membrane Ig, the exons for the transmembrane segments are spliced to a point just within the final C domain. If this does not occur, the stop signal is retained and mRNA for secreted Ig is produced. The point of polyadenylation controls how the primary transcript will be spliced. Initially, a B cell joins a μ gene to its VDJ gene, but other C genes may alternatively be linked to VDJ; this is called class switching.

Class switching is a process by which the cell can switch the class of Ig it produces while retaining the same antigen specificity. All the heavy-chain constant-region genes except D are preceded by a switching sequence. Switching is effected by bringing a new C gene up to the position occupied by the μ C gene, with the loss of the intervening C genes. This process is illustrated above for the switch from IgM to IgG1. It is also possible for a cell to switch classes by producing very long primary RNA transcripts, which are then spliced to connect the new C gene to VDJ. Indeed, this is the only way that IgD (which lacks a switch sequence) can be produced. This process is controlled by T cells and is modulated by cytokines. For example, IL-4 promotes switching to IgG1 and IgE in the mouse.

ANTIBODY FRAGMENTS

Much of the early work on the elucidation of antibody structure was performed using fragments of antibodies prepared by methods such as enzyme digestion and selective reduction of the disulphide bonds. Of particular interest are the Fab and F(ab')$_2$ fragments. Fab has one antigen-combining site and so cannot crosslink antigenic determinants, whereas F(ab')$_2$ has two sites and can crosslink. Lacking the Fc region, they are both useful in determining which antibody functions are Fc-dependent. The table below illustrates the structures of the fragments (yellow) and their means of production. IgG fragments are illustrated, but analogous fragments can be made from other classes of Igs. More recently, Fv fragments consisting of linked V$_H$ and V$_L$ domains have been produced by molecular biological techniques.

fragment	structure	produced by
F(ab')$_2$	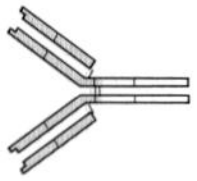	pepsin digestion
Fab'	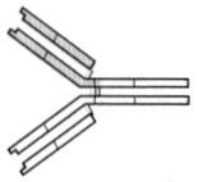	pepsin digestion and partial reduction
Fab	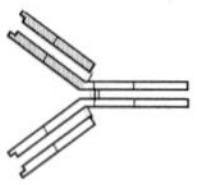	papain digestion
Fc	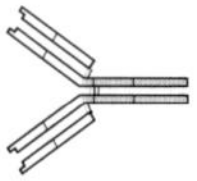	papain digestion
Facb	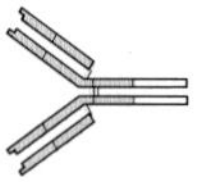	plasmin digestion
pFc'	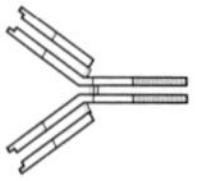	pepsin or plasmin digestion
Fd	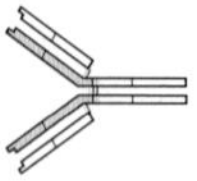	pepsin digestion partial reduction and reaggregation
Fv		molecular biology

Fig. 2.11 Antibody fragments.

ANTIGENS

Immunogens. An antigen is any molecule recognized by the immune system, but the term immunogen is reserved for those antigens which elicit a strong immune response, particularly in the context of protective immunity to pathogenic organisms.

Haptens and Carriers. Artificial antigens have been used to examine the immune response. In particular, small antigenic determinants (haptens) are covalently coupled to larger molecules (carriers). Haptens bind to antibodies but cannot by themselves elicit an antibody response. Haptens are recognized by B cells, which present fragments of the carriers to T cells.

T-dependent antigens need to be recognized by both T cells and B cells to elicit an antibody response. Most protein antigens fall into this category. Immune responses to T-dep antigens show class switching to IgG with an increase in antibody affinity.

T-independent antigens can stimulate B cells to produce antibody without T cell help. Most such antigens are large polymeric molecules with repeated epitopes, capable of crosslinking surface Ig, and are only slowly degraded.

Type I and II T-independent antigens are differentiated according to their ability to activate different B cell subsets. Type I antigens stimulate both Lyb5+ and Lyb5- cells (mouse), whereas type II antigens can only act on Lyb5+ cells.

antigen	polymer	B cell mitogen	resistance to degradation	type
lipopolysaccharide (LPS)	+	+ + +	+	1
PPD	−	+ + +	+	1
dextran	+ +	−	+ +	2
levan	+ +	−	+ +	2
Ficoll	+ + +	−	+ + +	2
polymerized flagellin	+ +	+	+	2
poly I: poly C	+ +	+ +	+	2
poly D amino acids	+ + +	−	+ + +	2

Fig. 2.12 Properties of commonly used T-independent antigens.

ANTIGEN/ANTIBODY INTERACTIONS

Epitopes and Paratopes are part of a nomenclature used to describe the interaction between antigen and antigen receptor molecules, including antibodies. An epitope is an antigenic determinant, and the paratope, formed by the hypervariable loops of the V domains, is the part of the antibody which binds to the epitope.

Contact residues are the amino acids of the epitope and paratope which contribute to the antigen/antibody bond.

Continuous and Discontinuous epitopes. Study of the precise molecular interaction between antigen and antibody shows that some epitopes are formed by one linear stretch of amino acids (continuous epitope). In most cases, however, an epitope has contact residues derived from different sections of a protein antigen, brought together by folding of the polypeptide chain (discontinuous epitope).

Antigen/antibody bond. Antibodies bind specifically to the antigen which induced their formation, by multiple non-covalent bonds, including Van der Waal's forces, salt bridges, hydrogen bonds and hydrophobic interactions. Crystallographic studies of immune complexes between antibodies and protein antigens indicate that they interact by complementary surfaces of up to 1000Å^2 with the third hypervariable regions (VJ and VDJ) lying near the centre of the binding site. Hypervariable regions of both L and H chains contribute contact residues. The diagram opposite (top) shows lysozyme antigen (green), and the light (yellow) and heavy (blue) chains of a complexed anti-lysozyme antibody. The lower diagram shows the molecules rotated forward 90°, with contact residues (red and pink) numbered on the interacting faces.

Charge neutralization refers to the observation that charged contact residues on an epitope are often neutralized by residues of an opposite charge on the paratope. This is particularly important at the centre of the binding site.

Induced fit refers to the flexing of residues in the hypervariable loops in contact with the epitope, which may occur to allow an optimum fit between the interacting molecules.

Antibody affinity is a measure of the bond strength between a single epitope and a paratope. It depends on the sum of the bond energies of the non-covalent interactions, set against the natural repulsion between molecules and the energy required to make any necessary distortions to allow binding (induced fit).

Antibody valency describes the number of binding sites on a molecule. For example, IgG has two sites and IgM has 10, although the effective number depends on the configuration of the antigen.

Antibody avidity is the total strength of an antigen/antibody bond, which is related to the affinity of the paratope/epitope bonds and antibody valency. Binding energy is much enhanced when several bonds form, so avidity usually exceeds affinity.

Cross-reaction. Some antisera are not totally specific for their inducing antigen but bind related (cross-reacting) antigens, either due to sharing a common epitope, or because the molecular shapes of the cross-reacting antigens are similar.

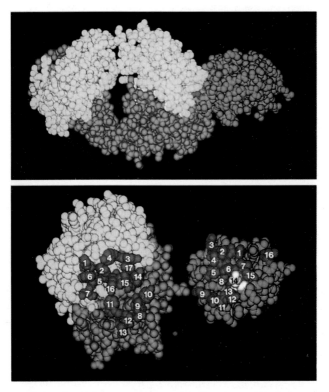

Fig. 2.13 The Fab/lysozyme complex. Courtesy of Dr R.J. Poljak from *Science* (1986) **233**, 747–753. Copyright 1986 by the AAAS.

T CELL ANTIGEN RECEPTOR (TCR)

The TCR consists of a heterodimer (Ti), and a number of associated polypeptides which form the CD3 complex. The dimer recognizes processed antigen associated with an MHC molecule. The CD3 complex is required for receptor expression and is involved in signal transduction.

TCR$\alpha\beta$ (TCR2) and TCR$\gamma\delta$ (TCR1). The polypeptide chains for the antigen-binding portion of the receptor are encoded by four different gene loci: α, β, γ and δ. Any T cell will express either an $\alpha\beta$ or a $\gamma\delta$ receptor. The great majority of thymocytes and peripheral T cells have a TCR$\alpha\beta$.

Ti is a term used to distinguish the antigen/MHC-binding portion (which differs between cells), from the monomorphic CD3 complex. The N-terminal domains of $\alpha\beta$ or $\gamma\delta$ resemble a membrane-bound Fab, with variable (V) domains forming the antigen/MHC receptor, and membrane-proximal constant (C) domains.

CD3 complex in man consists of four polypeptide chains, each of which spans the cell membrane. These are the γ, δ, ϵ and ζ chains. The first three are structurally related, single-domain members of the Ig supergene family, whereas the ζ chains are unrelated and form ζ–ζ dimers. In mice, a fifth chain, η, is also present as a minority alternative partner for ζ chains, making an η–ζ dimer. The CD3 ζ–ζ dimer has intracellular ITAM motifs, which become phosphorylated after the receptor binds to antigen/MHC, allowing it to bind kinases, which then initiate a cascade of activation steps.

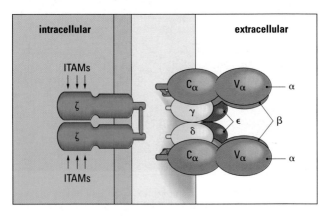

Fig. 2.14 A model of a T cell receptor complex (TCR2).

T CELL RECEPTOR GENES

The genes for the antigen/MHC-binding portion of the TCR are similar to those of antibody, in that they consist of multiple V, D and J segments which become recombined during T cell development to produce functional VDJ or VJ genes (see pp. 32–33). These encode the N-terminal variable (V) domains of the TCR. The α and γ loci have V and J segments only, whereas β and δ have V, D and J segments. The recombined V gene is linked to the exons for the C domains, the short hinge-like section (containing the inter-chain disulphide bond), the transmembrane and cytoplasmic segments. The layout of the human α and β loci are shown below, and that of the mouse α, γ and δ loci is very similar. Note that there are tandem sets of genes for the β-chain D, J and C regions. Each locus is distinct, although the δ-chain D, J and C genes lie between the V_α and J_α genes. The process of recombination can permit variability in the precise linking position of V to J, the possibility of linking the D segments in all three reading frames, and the addition of N-region diversity – ie. bases inserted into the junctions, which are not encoded in the germline. Theoretically, the arrangement of recombination sequences flanking the D_β and D_δ genes permits the assembly of genes with more than one D region (ie. VDDJ). In contrast to antibody genes, the TCR genes do not undergo somatic hypermutation. Nevertheless, the amount of diversity that can be generated is at least as great as for antibodies. The genes for the γ, δ and ϵ polypeptides of the CD3 complex do not undergo any rearrangements and are closely linked on chromosome 11 in man. All CD3 genes are required for TCR expression, and charged residues in the CD3 chain transmembrane segments are thought to be involved in association with antigen/MHC-binding $\alpha\beta$ or $\gamma\delta$ dimers.

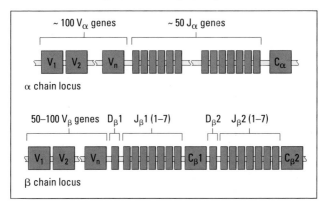

Fig. 2.15 Genes of the human *TCRA* (α) and *TCRB* (β) loci.

MHC MOLECULES

Major Histocompatibility Complex (MHC) is a large group of genes including those encoding the class I and II MHC molecules, which are involved in presentation of antigen to T cells. The complex was originally identified as a locus encoding allogeneic cell surface molecules involved in graft rejection. It is now known that MHC molecules are essential for presentation of antigen from within cells, to T cells.

MHC class I molecules are integral membrane proteins found on all nucleated cells and platelets. These are the classical transplantation antigens. They each have one polypeptide chain encoded within the MHC which traverses the plasma membrane. The extracellular portion has three domains (α_1–α_3). The membrane-proximal α_3 domain is associated with β_2-microglobulin, while the two N-terminal domains form an antigen-binding pocket consisting of a base of β-pleated sheet derived from both α_1 and α_2 domains surrounded by two loops of α-helix. Residues facing into the binding pocket vary between different molecules and haplotypes, to allow different antigenic peptides to bind. The α_3 domain has a binding site for CD8. There are several MHC class I-like molecules (functions unknown) encoded in the MHC or elsewhere, which are called non-classical MHC class I molecules.

β_2-Microglobulin is a polypeptide chain encoded by genes outside the MHC, which forms a single domain, related to Ig domains. It is necessary for loading and transport of class I molecules to the cell surface and their expression there.

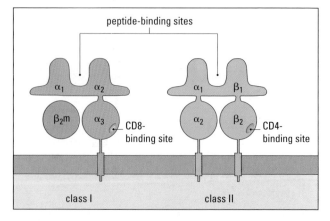

Fig. 2.16 Structures of MHC class I and class II molecules.

MHC class II molecules (Ia antigens) are expressed on B cells, macrophages, monocytes, APCs and some T cells. They consist of two non-covalently linked polypeptides (α and β), both encoded by the MHC, which traverse the plasma membrane, each having two extracellular domains. Class II molecules resemble class I molecules, with the N-terminal α_1 and β_1 domains forming the peptide binding site. A site in the β_2 domain binds to CD4.

MHC class III molecules are a variety of proteins, also encoded in the MHC. They include complement components (C4, C2, FB), heat shock proteins and cytokines. Also present are the LMP and TAP genes, the products of which are involved in the degradation and transport of antigenic peptides. The DM genes encode class II-like molecules which facilitate loading of class II molecules with antigenic peptides.

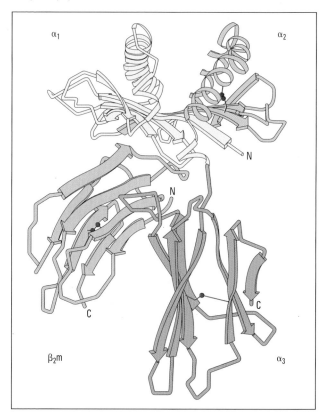

Fig. 2.17 Structure of a class I MHC molecule.

MHC GENES

H-2 is the mouse major histocompatibility complex, which lies on chromosome 17. There are six main regions: K, M, A, E, S and D. Genes with immunological functions in each of these regions are shown below. Pseudogenes have been omitted.

H-2K and H-2D encode class I MHC molecules, the classical transplantation antigens. The K locus has one gene, whereas the number of genes in the D locus varies between strains.
H-2M encodes a class II molecule involved in antigen processing and is analogous to DM in man.
LMP gene products are components of proteasomes.
TAP gene products transport antigen fragments.
H-2A and H-2E (I-A and I-E) encode the α and β chains of the class II molecules. This was previously designated the H-2I region and subdivided into I-A and I-E.
H-2S contains genes for the complement components C2, factor B (Bf) and C4, as well as the cytokines TNF-α and TNF-β.
Slp (sex-limited protein) is a non-functional variant of C4.
Qa and Tla loci lie downstream of the H-2 complex and contain genes for more than 25 class IV genes (non-classical class I genes). They may function as haemopoietic differentiation molecules, but may also be a source of DNA for gene conversion with conventional class I molecules.

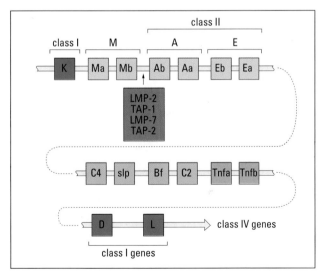

Fig. 2.18 H-2 – the mouse major histocompatibility complex.

HLA (Human Leucocyte Antigen) locus is the human major histocompatibility complex, and is divided into eight main regions: DP, DM, DQ, DR, class III, B, C and A. It is thought that a number of class IV genes lie downstream of HLA-A. The overall layout is very similar to that of the mouse H-2 region.

HLA-A, -B and -C loci encode class I MHC. The A and B loci show greatest polymorphism, with 99 and 50 haplotypes, respectively, whereas 34 have been defined at the C locus.

HLA-DP, -DQ and -DR loci encode class II MHC molecules. Originally these were described as HLA-D specificities, detected by their ability to stimulate allogeneic cells in a mixed lymphocyte culture (MLC). Now the different molecules are defined serologically, although this can only be partly related to their HLA-D designation. DP and DQ each encode one pair of class II α and β chains, plus pseudogenes. The DR locus encodes one non-polymorphic α chain and 1–4 β chains, depending on the individual haplotype.

HLA-DM encodes the class II molecule DM, which is involved in loading peptides onto class II molecules.

HLA class III molecules are encoded between the class II loci and the class I loci. They include the C2 and factor B genes and the pseudoalleles for C4, C4F and C4S, which determine the Rogers and Chido blood groups, respectively. Genes for TNF-α, TNF-β and some heat shock proteins also lie here.

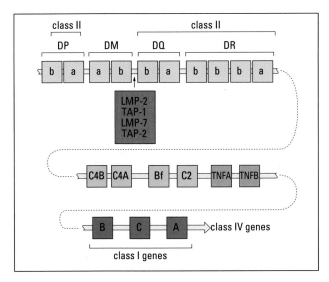

Fig. 2.19 HLA – the human major histocompatibility complex.

Immune Responses | 3

ADAPTIVE AND INNATE IMMUNITY

The immune response is mediated by a variety of cells and soluble factors, broadly divided according to whether they mediate adaptive (acquired) or innate (natural) immunity.

Adaptive (Acquired) immunity is specific for the inducing agent, and is marked by an enhanced response on repeated encounters with that agent. Thus the key features of the adaptive immune response are *memory* and *specificity*.

Innate (Natural) immunity depends on a variety of immunological effector mechanisms, which are neither specific for particular infectious agents nor improved by repeated encounters with the same agent. In practice, there is considerable overlap between these two types of immunity, since the adaptive immune system can direct elements of the innate system, such as phagocytes or complement. The principal elements of the innate immune system are outlined below.

Complement system is a group of serum molecules involved in the control of inflammation, removal of immune complexes and lysis of pathogens or cells sensitized with antibody.

Acute phase proteins describes those serum molecules which increase rapidly at the onset of infection. The most notable is C-reactive protein (CRP), which binds the C-protein of *Pneumococcus* spp. and facilitates their uptake by phagocytes.

	innate immune system	adaptive immune system
	resistance not improved by repeated infection	resistance improved by repeated infection
soluble factors	lysozyme, complement, acute phase proteins eg. CRP, interferon	antibody
cells	phagocytes natural killer (NK) cells	T lymphocytes

Fig. 3.1 Elements of the innate and adaptive immune systems.

Interferons (IFNs) are a group of molecules which limit the spread of viral infections. There are three types: IFN-α and IFN-β, produced by leucocytes and fibroblasts, and IFN-γ, produced by activated T cells. IFNs from activated or virally infected cells bind to receptors on nearby cells, inducing them to make anti-viral proteins. IFN-α and IFN-β bind to one type of receptor, while IFN-γ binds to another. IFN-γ also has many other immunomodulatory functions.

Anti-viral proteins are molecules that are induced by IFNs, which limit viral replication. Many of them are produced in an inactive form, and are only activated by contact with the virus or its products, such as double-stranded RNA. Some, activated by an incoming virus, block the initiation of protein synthesis, whereas others lead to mRNA degradation.

Cell-mediated immunity and Humoral immunity are traditional ways of describing the different arms of the immune system. Antibody, complement and other soluble molecules constitute the humoral effector systems, whereas T cells, NK cells and phagocytes constitute the cellular effectors. With advances in our understanding of immune recognition, it is more useful to think in terms of the systems that recognize free antigens, and those that recognize cell-associated antigens. For example, cytotoxic T cells can recognize antigens presented on cell membranes which have originated from within that cell, whereas antibody is particularly important in the recognition of free, extracellular antigens.

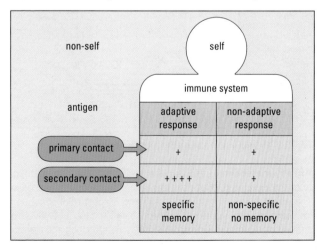

Fig. 3.2 Primary and secondary immune responses.

ANTIBODY RESPONSE

Following injection of an antigen, an antibody response develops which may be divided into four phases: a lag phase in which no antibody is detected, followed by a phase in which the antibody titres rise logarithmically, then plateau and decline, as the antibodies are catabolized or cleared as complexes.

Primary and Secondary antibody responses. The quality of the antibody response following the second (secondary) encounter with antigen varies from that following the first (primary) contact. The primary response has a longer lag phase, reaches a lower plateau and declines more quickly than the secondary response. IgM is a major component of the primary response and is produced before IgG, whereas IgG is the main class represented in the secondary response. During their development, some B cells switch from IgM production to other classes, and this is the basis of the change in antibody isotype seen in the secondary response. Differences between the primary and secondary response are most noticeable when T-dependent antigens are used, but the route of antigen entry and the way it is presented to T and B cells also affect the development of the response and the classes of antibody produced.

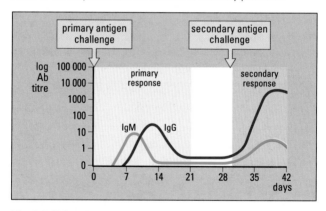

Fig. 3.3 Primary and secondary antibody responses.

Affinity maturation describes the finding that the average affinity of the induced antibodies increases in the secondary response. The effect is largely confined to IgG and is most marked when a low antigen dose is given in the secondary injection. Low levels of antigen bind preferentially to high-affinity B cell clones and activate them – there is insufficient antigen to activate low-affinity clones. The underlying cellular basis is the change in the affinity of B cell

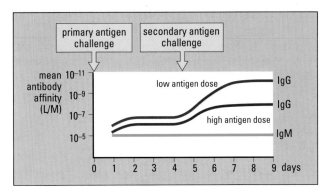

Fig. 3.4 Affinity maturation.

clones, caused by somatic hypermutation of the antibody genes which occurs in the germinal centres, where B cells compete for antigen on follicular dendritic cells. The process is accompanied by, but is not dependent on, class switching. It does not occur in the response to T-independent antigens, which are predominantly IgM antibodies. Therefore the survival and development of high-affinity B cells depends on T cells.

Active immunization/Vaccination are the terms used for the active induction of protective immunity against a pathogen. It depends on the greater effectiveness of the secondary immune response. Vaccines may be live attenuated organisms, killed organisms, individual antigens of a pathogen, or modified antigens. In general, living organisms are more effective than killed ones or individual antigens, except in the case of diseases where the pathology is caused by a toxin (eg. diphtheria). In this case, a mod-ified toxin, or toxoid, which retains antigenicity but lacks patho-genicity is preferred. Newer vaccines may be made by genetic engineering. For example, genes for antigens of pathogenic virus-es such as hepatitis can be inserted into non-pathogenic viruses such as vaccinia. It is also possible to insert small fragments of antigens, which are known to act as T cell epitopes, into such car-rier viruses. One limitation of this approach, however, is that dif-ferent peptides are presented by different MHC molecules, so a peptide which is antigenic in one individual may not be in another.

Passive immunization is the administration of antibodies pre-formed in another individual, to contribute to protective immunity against a pathogen. It is used when an individual's own active response would be too slow, for example in producing a response to snake venoms or tetanus toxoid.

CELL COOPERATION

Cooperation between cells involved in immune responses occurs at many levels. Dendritic cells can take up antigen in the periphery and transport it to secondary lymphoid tissues (spleen, lymph nodes etc.) for presentation to T cells. B cells and macrophages can also internalize antigen, process it and present it in association with MHC class II molecules to CD4+ TH cells. Cytokines produced by activated TH2 cells stimulate B cell growth and differentiation into plasma cells. Other cytokines can also activate Tc cells, APCs and mononuclear phagocytes. Antibodies released by the B cells can bind to receptors on phagocytes, thereby facilitating uptake of antigen. IgG antibodies allow LGLs (K cells) to recognize target cells coated with antibody, and IgE antibodies can sensitize mast cells and basophils to release their inflammatory mediators when they bind specific antigen. Cytokines and antibodies are soluble mediators of cell cooperation, but leucocytes also interact directly with each other. The most important direct interaction is that involving MHC molecules/antigenic peptides contacting the T cell receptor, but other interactions are essential for cellular cooperation, including adhesion and costimulation.

Antigen presentation is the process by which antigen is presented to lymphocytes in a form they can recognize. Most CD4+ T cells must be presented with antigen on MHC class II molecules, while CD8+ Tc cells only recognize antigen on class I MHC molecules. Antigen must be processed into peptide fragments before it can associate with MHC molecules. The way in which an antigen is processed and the type of MHC molecule it associates with determine which T cells will recognize it and whether the antigen is immunogenic or tolerogenic, and affect the type of immune response generated.

Adhesion is an essential component of the interactions between leucocytes and other cells. It controls the position of a cell in lymphoid tissue, controls migration into tissues and is aprerequisite for antigen presentation and many immune effector functions.

Costimulation. Most immune responses are initiated by antigen triggering B cells or T cells. However, cellular activation also requires other signals. These may be delivered via costimulatory molecules (eg. CD40 for B cells or CD28 for T cells) or by cytokines. This is sometimes called the two-signal hypothesis, in which antigen provides the first signal and the other costimulatory interactions provide the second signal. Cells which only receive a first signal may become anergic (tolerant) to their particular antigen.

Cytokines (Lymphokines) are a group of molecules, other than antibodies, produced by leucocytes, which are involved in signalling between cells of the immune system. The group includes the interleukins, the interferons, the tumour necrosis factors (TNFs) and the colony-stimulating factors (CSFs). The term lymphokines was originally used for those cytokines produced by lymphocytes.

T cell help describes the cooperative interactions between TH2 cells and B cells in the production of the antibody response to T-dep antigens, or between TH1 cells and macrophages in cell-mediated responses. In either case, the B cell or macrophage presents processed antigen to the T cell, receives costimulatory signals and is then triggered by specific cytokines. For example, a B cell internalizes its own specific antigen and presents it to the T cell. It transduces costimulatory signals via CD40, and is further activated by the cytokines IL-4, IL-2, IL-13 and IL-6.

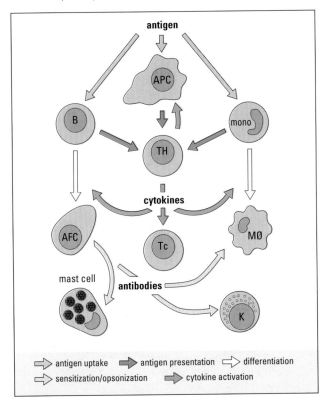

Fig. 3.5 Cooperation between cells in the immune response.

ANTIGEN PRESENTATION

Antigens are taken up by antigen-presenting cells in a variety of ways. B cells use surface antibody to bind and internalize their specific antigen. This is partly degraded (processed) and returned to the cell surface, associated with MHC class II molecules, for recognition by TH2 cells. Theoretically, B cells can endocytose and present any antigen, but in practice they selectively concentrate only their own specific antigen in sufficient quantities. Mononuclear phagocytes endocytose opsonized particles via their Fc and C3 receptors, which are partly degraded before presentation to TH1 cells. How dendritic cells handle antigen is less well understood, since their ability to endocytose antigen is limited. They may endocytose and degrade sufficient material themselves, before they enter the lymphoid tissue, or they may take up antigens that have been degraded by other cells.

Antigen processing is the process of antigen breakdown and its association with MHC molecules. Blocking degradative pathways leaves cells unable to process and present most antigens. Different cell types have different capacities to degrade antigens, and hence different abilities to stimulate T cells. There are two distinct pathways for antigen processing, used by MHC class I and class II molecules. These are referred to as the internal and external pathways, since MHC class I presents antigens from inside the cell, while MHC class II presents antigens which the cell has endocytosed.

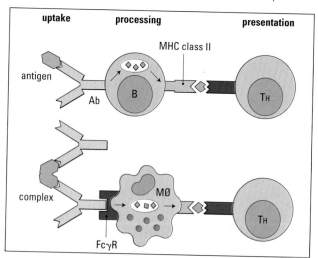

Fig. 3.6 Antigen processing and presentation by APCs.

Class II (External) pathway. Antigens such as immune complexes that have been endocytosed by a cell, associate preferentially with MHC class II molecules. The endocytosed antigens are partly degraded, and the endocytic vesicles containing peptide fragments then fuse with vesicles containing MHC class II molecules.

Invariant chain (Ii, CD74). MHC class II molecules are initially produced in association with an invariant chain, Ii, which is required for folding of the MHC class II molecule and prevents peptides binding to the class II in the endoplasmic reticulum. The invariant chain targets MHC class II to the MIIC compartment.

MIIC compartment is an acidic endosomal compartment where antigenic peptide fragments and MHC class II molecules combine. The invariant chain is degraded, leaving a small peptide, CLIP, bound to the class II molecule. Once this has been replaced by an antigenic peptide, the class II/antigen complex can be finally processed before moving to the cell surface.

Antigenic peptides are the protein fragments which bind to MHC molecules. Class I molecules accommodate nine amino acids in their peptide-binding groove; class II molecules 12–15 amino acids.

DM molecules are class II-like molecules which are required to facilitate loading of peptides onto the class II molecules.

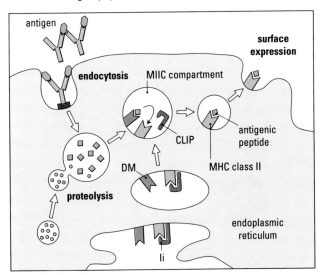

Fig. 3.7 Antigen presentation: MHC class II pathway.

Class I (Internal) pathway. Antigens synthesized within a cell, such as viral polypeptides, and the cell's own proteins associate preferentially with MHC class I molecules. Peptide fragments from the cytosol are sampled for review by CD8+ T cells.

Proteasomes are multicatalytic protease complexes which break down cytosolic proteins into fragments. Two components of the proteasome (LMP-2 and LMP-7) are encoded within the MHC. Proteasomes generate antigen fragments which may be loaded onto MHC class I molecules.

TAP-1 and TAP-2 are MHC-encoded members of the ABC family of transporters. They transfer peptides across the membrane of the endoplasmic reticulum, to be presented by MHC class I molecules.

MHC class I/antigen assembly takes place in the endoplasmic reticulum. Peptide fragments associate with the α chain of the class I molecule, which is then stabilized by β_2-microglobulin. Complexes which do not assemble correctly are degraded, while class I molecules loaded with peptides are transported to the cell surface.

Anchor residues are critical amino acids required for an antigenic peptide to bind to an MHC molecule. Class I molecules bind nonapeptides with dominant anchor positions at residues 2, 5 and 9. The requirement for particular amino acids at each position depends on the haplotype of the MHC molecule.

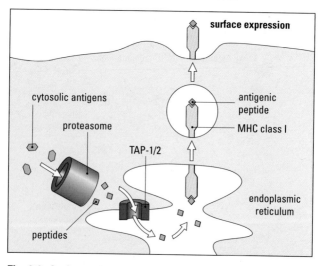

Fig. 3.8 Antigen presentation: MHC class I pathway.

MHC restriction. T cells recognize antigen associated with particular MHC molecules. For example, a T cell that recognizes an antigen associated with H-2K^b will not recognize it associated with H-2D^b or H-2K^k. Such interactions are MHC restricted. The basis of the observation is that T cells that interact with self MHC molecules are selectively expanded in the thymus, and are then primed to respond to antigen on APCs expressing these MHC molecules. Subsequently, they will respond only to that antigen/MHC combination. Experimentally, it is possible to determine whether an immune interaction involves MHC molecules by seeing whether it is MHC restricted.

Class I/class II restriction refers to whether a particular group of T cells recognize antigen associated with MHC class I or class II molecules. In practice, CD8$^+$ cells are class I restricted, whereas CD4$^+$ cells are class II restricted.

CD4 and CD8 are functionally analogous molecules expressed on mature T cells. The cells have either CD4 or CD8 but not both. CD8 consists of two disulphide-linked transmembrane polypeptides, which can interact with the TCR on the T cells and which bind to a site in the α_3 domain of class I MHC molecules on the target cell (see below). This interaction contributes to the stabilization of the immune recognition complex. CD4 has a single transmembrane polypeptide chain and binds MHC class II on APCs. The kinase lck, associated with CD4, phosphorylates the TCR after antigen/MHC binding.

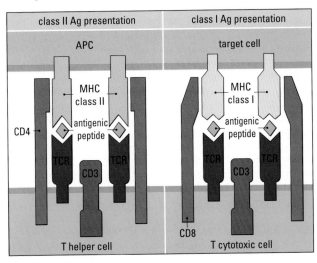

Fig. 3.9 Immune recognition by T cells.

T CELL ACTIVATION

T cells require three types of signal for full activation:
- Antigenic peptide presented on an MHC molecule.
- Costimulatory signals.
- Signalling by specific cytokines.

If a cell does not receive a full set of signals, it will not divide, and may even become anergic. Molecules such as CD2 and LFA-1 contribute to the adhesion between a T cell and an APC and enhance activation signals, but costimulation transduced via CD28 is essential for activation.

CD2 (Sheep erythrocyte receptor) is expressed on all T cells, and is involved in T cell activation. It has a single transmembrane polypeptide chain, which acts as a receptor for LFA-3 (CD58). Interaction of CD2 with LFA-3 enhances the binding of the T cell to its target. T cells can be activated by crosslinking their CD2 molecules, but it is thought that the normal function is to amplify an activation signal initiated by the TCR/CD3 complex. CD48 in rodents acts as an alternate ligand for CD2. Cell activation via CD2 causes phosphorylation of CD33 and CD37.

Lymphocyte Functional Antigen-3 (LFA-3, CD58), the receptor for CD2, is a two-domain member of the Ig superfamily, widely distributed on many cell types, which contributes to lymphocyte activation by crosslinking CD2.

Lymphocyte Functional Antigen-1 (LFA-1, CD11a/18) is a member of the β_2 integrin family present on most leucocytes. It consists of two polypeptide chains (CD11a and CD18), which interact with the adhesion molecules ICAM-1, ICAM-2 and ICAM-3. Transient adhesion between lymphocytes and APCs may be mediated by LFA-1 adhering to ICAM-1 and ICAM-3. Lymphocyte activation enhances the affinity of LFA-1, thereby increasing the strength of lymphocyte binding. Binding to ICAM-1 or ICAM-3 also contributes to T cell activation. Interaction of LFA-1 with ICAM-1 is important in the attachment of lymphocytes to endothelium prior to migration into sites of inflammation, since ICAM-1 is induced on endothelium by inflammatory cytokines. LFA-1 also binds to ICAM-2, which is expressed constitutively on endothelium but not on other cell types.

ICAM-3 (CD50) is present on many leucocytes, although expression is increased following lymphocyte activation. It contributes to T cell interactions with APCs.

CD28 and CTLA-4 are molecules which critically regulate T cell activation. CD28 is present on 80% of CD4 T cells and 50% (approx.) of CD8 cells. The molecule B7, expressed on many APCs, is the principal ligand for CD28. Ligation of CD28 is an essential costimulatory signal for T cell activation. CD28 is down-regulated after activation. By contrast, CTLA-4, an alternative ligand for B7 which is not expressed on resting T cells, is induced after T cell activation at the time when CD28 expression is reduced. Ligation of CD28 may act by rescuing cells from apoptosis, but it also plays a role in promoting a TH2 type of response: CD28 knockout mice have reduced antibody responses to some viruses, while the TH1 response is intact. The role of CTLA-4 is less clear, but it appears to counter some of the costimulatory effects of CD28 and this may be due to competition for B7.

B7-1 (CD80) and B7-2 (CD86) are ligands for CD28 and CTLA-4, induced on B cells following stimulation with LPS, binding of antigen to surface Ig, or B cell activation by CD40 or IL-4. By contrast, crosslinking of B cell Fc receptors reduces B7 expression. B7 is also inducible on mononuclear phagocytes, by LPS or IFN-γ, and is constitutively expressed on dendritic cells.

IL-2 Receptor (IL-2R, CD25) is induced on stimulated T cells. The high-affinity receptor is formed when the induced α chain (CD25) associates with the β and γ chains, which alone form a low-affinity receptor. IL-2 is essential for cell division and the high-affinity receptor persists for several days after T cell activation.

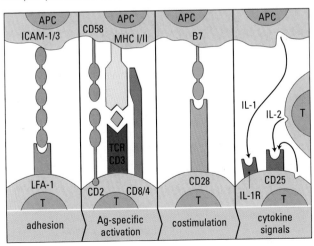

Fig. 3.10 Steps in T cell activation.

B CELL ACTIVATION

B cells responding to T-dependent antigens require three types of signal for their activation. The first signal is mediated by the binding of antigen, which is processed and presented to T cells. Then a costimulatory signal is transduced via CD40, which is ligated by CD40L. Thereafter, B cell division, differentiation and Ig class switching are driven by a large number of different cytokines. Type-2 T-independent antigens such as polysaccharides that crosslink B cell surface antibody can activate B cells directly, although such B cells still need cytokine signals.

Intermolecular help refers to the way in which B cells taking up antigenic particles carrying several different antigens (eg. a virus) can then present the entire set of antigens to T cells. They thus get help from T cells recognizing antigens that they themselves do not.

CD40 is a surface protein present on B cells, follicular dendritic cells, dendritic cells, macrophages, endothelium and haemopoietic progenitors. It belongs to the TNF receptor family. It provides a critical costimulatory signal to B cells, but is also involved in thymocyte selection and induction of peripheral tolerance.

CD40L (gp39) is the ligand for CD40, induced transiently on CD4+ T cells and some CD8 cells following activation. It is also present on eosinophils and basophils. CD40L is essential for delivery of T cell help to B cells. Absence of CD40L in X-linked hyper-IgM syn-

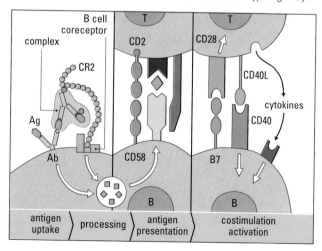

Fig. 3.11 Steps in B cell activation.

drome results in a failure of B cell class switching. It is also needed for the development of germinal centres and B cell memory.

CD45 (Leucocyte common antigen) is a phosphatase present on all leucocytes and is produced in six different forms, using combinations of exons. B cells express the highest molecular weight form. It is thought to be involved in the early stages of cell activation, by controlling phosphorylation of molecules such as CD4.

B cell coreceptor complex (CD19, CD21/CR2, CD81/TAPA-1) amplifies signalling via the antigen receptor on B cells. Crosslinking of CD19 to surface Ig makes a B cell 100× more sensitive to antigen. This is important in the initial development of an antibody response when the B cell antibody is of low affinity. Immune complexes formed in the primary immune response may fix complement C3, and this can then bind to CD21 on the B cell which is complement receptor type 2 (CR2). If the complexed antigen is recognized by the B cell antigen receptor, the complex crosslinks the coreceptor complex and surface Ig, thereby activating the B cell very efficiently. This may explain the long-standing observation that complement is required for development of secondary antibody responses and B cell memory.

CD23 (FcεRII) is a low-affinity receptor for IgE with a lectin domain, but it is also an alternative ligand for CR2 (see above). It is expressed on B cells, activated macrophages and follicular dendritic cells, but may also be released in a soluble form to act as a costimulatory factor in B cell activation.

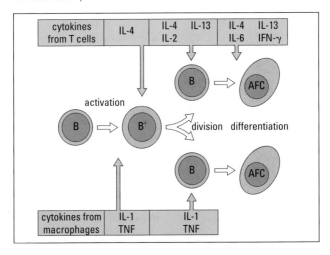

Fig. 3.12 Role of cytokines in B cell development.

CYTOKINES

Cytokines, released by leucocytes and sometimes other cells, are very important in controlling the development of the immune response. They modulate the differentiation and division of haemopoietic stem cells and the activation of lymphocytes and phagocytes. They control the balance between cell-mediated immune responses and antibody production. Others can act as mediators of inflammation or as cytotoxins. Many cytokines have more than one action (pleiotropy) and different cells produce different blends of cytokines. The ability to respond to any particular cytokine depends on the expression of a specific receptor. Often more than one cytokine signal is required for a response and in this case the different cytokines act synergistically. T helper cells are particularly important sources of cytokines.

Autocrine and Paracrine actions. Most cytokines act on cells other than those that produced them (paracrine action), but some can also stimulate the cell that produced them (autocrine action).

Interleukins (IL-1–IL-17) are a series of diverse cytokines; most newly discovered cytokines are placed in this series. Their principal properties are indicated opposite. IL-1 has many effects similar to TNF, including enhancing leucocyte/endothelial cell adhesion and inducing acute phase proteins. It can also act on hypothalamic centres to induce fever and sleep. It causes fibroblasts, osteoclasts and chondrocytes to produce prostaglandins and promote tissue remodelling. IL-1 induces IL-2 receptors on T cells and therefore acts as a costimulator in T cell activation. IL-2 is an essential T cell growth factor (TCGF) required for division of antigen-activated T cells. Activated B cells also express IL-2 receptors. IL-15 has functional similarities with IL-2. IL-3 is a pan-specific haemopoietin, while IL-7 is required for the development of pre-B cells and pre-T cells (see p. 17). IL-11 synergizes with IL-3 in haematopoiesis. IL-4 and IL-13 are essential B cell growth factors, while IL-6 promotes their subsequent differentiation into antibody-forming cells. IL-6 also has various proinflammatory actions. IL-4 tends to promote class switching to IgG2a (in mouse), whereas IFN-γ promotes IgG1 production. IL-5 also promotes B cell differentiation in some species but is essential for the differentiation of eosinophils. IL-9, in contrast, is important in mast cell differentiation. IL-8 is a chemokine released by activated monocytes which is chemotactic for neutrophils and basophils and causes monocytes to adhere to endothelium. IL-10, produced by TH2 cells, suppresses cytokine production by TH1 cells, thereby controlling the TH1/TH2 balance. IL-12 promotes TH1-type immune responses.

cytokine	source	target	principal effects
IL-1α	macrophage fibroblast lymphocytes	lymphocytes macrophages endothelium	lymphocyte costimulation phagocyte activation ↑ endothelial adhesion molecules
IL-1β	epithelial cells astrocytes	other	induces fever and sleep ↑ prostaglandin synthesis
IL-2	T cells	T cells NK cells B cells	T cell growth and activation NK cell activation division
IL-3	T cells thymic epithelium	stem cells	multi-lineage haemopoietic factor
IL-4	TH2 cells bone marrow stroma	B cells	activation and division promotes class switch → IgG1 and IgE
IL-5	TH2 cells	eosinophils B cells	development and differentiation
IL-6	macrophages endothelium TH2 cells	T cells B cells hepatocytes	lymphocyte growth B cell differentiation acute phase protein synthesis
IL-7	bone marrow stroma	pre-B cells pre-T cells	division
IL-8	fibroblasts monocytes endothelium	monocytes T cells neutrophils	activation/chemotaxis
IL-9	CD4 T cells	T cells mast cells	division promotes development
IL-10	TH2 cells	TH1 cells	inhibits cytokine synthesis
IL-11	bone marrow stroma	stem cells plasma cells	division proliferation
IL-12	B cells macrophages	TH0 cells NK cells	TH1 cell development activation
IL-13	TH2 cells	B cells macrophage	division and differentiation ↓ cytokine production
IL-14	T cells	B cells	proliferation ↓ Ig synthesis
IL-15	monocytes	T cells B cells	division
IL-16	CD8+ T cells	CD4+ T cells	chemotactic
IL-17	T cells	many cells	proinflammatory

Fig. 3.13 The interleukins.

Interferon-γ (IFN-γ) is released by antigen-activated TH1 cells. In addition to its antiviral effects, IFN-γ can enhance MHC class I and II expression on B cells and macrophages, and at higher levels induces class II on many tissue cells to enhance antigen presentation. It increases IL-2 receptors on Tc cells, enhances cytotoxic activity of NK cells and promotes B cell differentiation, favouring class switching to IgG2a in mice. IFN-γ is the principal cytokine responsible for 'Macrophage-Arming Factor' (MAF) activity, which increases FcγR expression and induces the respiratory burst, thereby enhancing their ability to destroy pathogens. It also inhibits TH2 cells, and so reinforces TH1-type immune responses.

Migration Inhibition Factor (MIF) is released by activated T cells and inhibits macrophage migration. It is important in causing the accumulation of these cells at sites of inflammation.

Tumour Necrosis Factor (TNF) and Lymphotoxin (LT-α) are structurally related cytokines encoded within the MHC. Lymphotoxin, released by Tc cells, is also called TNF-β, whereas the original TNF, released by activated macrophages and several other cell types, is TNF-α. A transmembrane form of lymphotoxin (LT-β), also produced by T cells, trimerizes with LT-α. In addition to its cytotoxic activity, TNF enhances the adhesiveness of vascular endothelium for leucocytes, by inducing E-selectin and ICAM-1 and thereby promoting transendothelial migration. The induction of acute phase protein synthesis by liver in response to TNF is probably mediated via IL-6. TNF also causes the mobilization of fat, which is partly responsible for the wasting (cachexia) seen in some chronic diseases. It also synergizes with IFN-γ in many of its actions, such as MHC induction and macrophage activation.

Transforming Growth Factor-β (TGF-β) is a group of five cytokines released by many cell types, including macrophages and platelets. They are mitogenic for fibroblasts and some other mesenchymal cells, and enhance the production of extracellular matrix proteins. In general, TGF-β is strongly inhibitory of immune responses, as it prevents proliferation of both T cells and B cells, and appears to be essential in controlling immune reactivity – TGF knockout mice develop severe and chronic inflammatory reactions.

Chemokines are a large group of small cytokines involved in activation of leucocytes during transendothelial migration (see p. 77), and in chemotaxis within tissues. The group includes IL-8, PF4, MCP-1, MIP-1α, MIP-1β and RANTES. They are selective for particular cell types and appear to control the phased arrival of different cell populations at sites of inflammation.

CYTOKINE RECEPTORS

Cytokine receptors determine the responsiveness of a cell to particular cytokines. Receptors for IL-1, TNF and the interferons are widely distributed. Others are induced on particular lineages for limited periods. For example, the high-affinity IL-2 receptor consists of three polypeptide chains, which appear together on antigen-activated T cells for a limited period, thereby controlling T cell division, but expression wanes if the T cell is not restimulated with antigen. Expression of receptors for IL-4 occurs on activated B cells in an analogous fashion. Receptors for colony-stimulating factors appear during haemopoietic cell differentiation on the appropriate developing cells. The cytokine receptors fall into families on the basis of structural motifs and shared chains. For example, the receptors for IL-2, IL-4, IL-7, IL-9 and IL-15 have a common signalling polypeptide (CD122) but individual cytokine-binding chains. IL-3 and IL-5 receptors share a different chain.

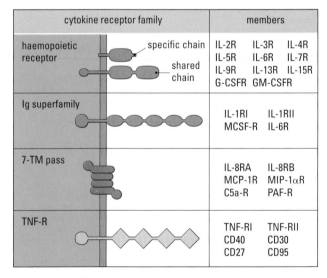

Fig. 3.14 Families of cytokine receptors.

Soluble cytokine receptors and cytokine inhibitors. Several cytokine receptors are produced in a soluble, truncated form, lacking the membrane-spanning domains. Examples are soluble TNF-R, IFN-γR and IL-1R. They are thought to limit the effects and zone of action of cytokines *in vivo*. Cytokine inhibitors have also been identified. For example, IL-1RA (IL-1 receptor antagonist) binds to the IL-1 receptor but does not activate the cell.

PHAGOCYTOSIS

Phagocytosis/endocytosis is the process by which cells engulf particles and microorganisms. The particles first attach to the cell membrane of the phagocytic cell, either by general receptors such as the mannosyl fucosyl receptor, which bind bacterial carbohydrates, or by receptors for specific opsonins such as IgG and C3b. Then the cell extends pseudopodia around the particle and internalizes it. Antibacterial oxygen-dependent killing mechanisms are activated, and lysosomes fuse with the phagosome. The lysosomal enzymes damage and digest the phagocytosed material and digestion products are finally released. Endocytosis is a general term which includes phagocytosis and pinocytosis (internalization of fluid).

Opsonization occurs when particles, microorganisms or immune complexes become coated with molecules which allow them to bind to receptors on phagocytes, thereby enhancing their uptake.

Opsonins are molecules which bind to particles to be phagocytosed and to receptors on phagocytes, so acting as a bridge between the two, eg. IgG, C3b and C-reactive protein.

Immune adherence, effected by IgG and C3 products, refers to the attachment of opsonized particles to phagocytes binding to Fc and complement receptors (see pp. 68 and 69).

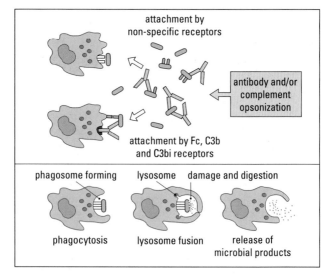

Fig. 3.15 Stages of phagocytosis.

Frustrated phagocytosis occurs when phagocytes attach to material which cannot be phagocytosed (eg. basement membrane). The cells may release their lysosomal enzymes to the exterior (exocytosis). This process is thought to cause some of the damage in immune complex diseases.

Phagosomes are the membrane-bound intracellular vesicles which contain phagocytosed materials.

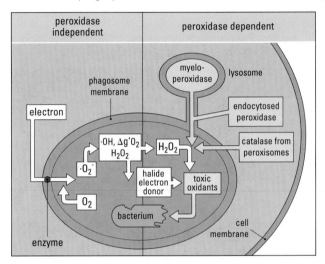

Fig. 3.16 Oxygen-dependent microbicidal activity.

Oxygen-dependent killing occurs within phagosomes and is activated via crosslinking of the phagocytes' C3 and Fc receptors. Initially, an enzyme, NADPH oxidase, is assembled in the phagosome membrane which reduces oxygen to superoxide (O_2^-) that can then give rise to hydroxyl radicals (OH^-), singlet oxygen ($O \cdot$) and hydrogen peroxide (H_2O_2).

Reactive Oxygen Intermediates (ROIs) refer to the labile products of the oxygen-dependent killing pathway (Fig. 3.16), which can damage endocytosed bacteria. Cells prevent damage to themselves by redox pathways involving glutathione, but some bacteria deploy similar defences against ROIs.

Myeloperoxidase present in lysosomes can enter the phagosome, where, in the presence of H_2O_2, it converts halide ions into toxic halogen compounds (eg. hypohalite). Endocytosed peroxidase or catalase can also perform this reaction.

Respiratory burst. Shortly after phagocytosing material, neutrophils and macrophages undergo a burst of activity, during which they increase their oxygen consumption. This is associated with increased activity of the hexose monophosphate shunt and production of H_2O_2 and $O_2\cdot$.

Reactive Nitrogen Intermediates (RNIs). Murine macrophages that have been activated by IFN-γ and triggered by TNF express a newly formed nitric oxide synthetase which catalyses the production of nitric oxide, NO, which is toxic for some bacteria and fungal pathogens. Although human macrophages do not produce significant amounts of NO, other cells (eg. neutrophils) can do so.

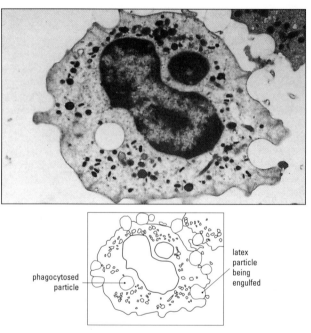

Fig. 3.17 Phagocytosis of latex by macrophages.

Lysosomes are organelles present in all cells. They contain enzymes which, in macrophages, damage and digest the phagocytosed material. Newly forming lysosomes are called 'primary' and mature lysosomes are 'secondary'.

Phagolysosomes are formed by the fusion of phagosomes and lysosomes. Immediately after phagosome/lysosome fusion, there is a brief rise in the pH of the phagolysosome, and neutral proteases and cationic proteins are active. Subsequently, the pH falls and acid proteases become active.

Granules are specialized lysosomes of granulocytes which contain various bactericidal proteins. Each type of granule has a particular set of proteins. For example, neutrophil myeloperoxidase is in the primary (azurophilic) granules, whereas lactoferrin is in the secondary (neutrophil specific) granules.

Granule and lysosome contents are listed below:

Lysozyme (Muramidase) is an enzyme which digests a bond in the cell wall proteoglycan of some Gram-positive bacteria. It is secreted constitutively by neutrophils and some macrophages and is present in many of the body's secretions.

Cationic proteins, found in neutrophil granules and in some macrophages, damage the outer lipid bilayer of some Gram-negative bacteria under alkaline conditions. This activity is produced by a number of molecules, some of which (eg. cathepsin G) are enzymically active.

Defensins are a group of small antimicrobial cytotoxic peptides present in neutrophil granules. They are most effective at alkaline pH – ie. they are cationic proteins. They have a wide spectrum of antibacterial and antifungal actions. Some defensins form ion channels in the target membrane; others interfere with metabolism.

Acid proteases are active at acid pH, and include enzymes such as glycosidase, nuclease, lipase and acid phosphatase.

Neutral proteases are active near pH 7, and include enzymes such as collagenase, elastase and some cathepsins.

Lactoferrin is found in neutrophil granules. It binds tightly to iron, thus depriving bacteria of this essential element. Neutrophils loaded with iron are inefficient at destroying bacteria.

Macrophage activation refers to the enhanced antimicrobial (or anti-tumour) activity seen in response to stimulation by cytokines, complement fragments and some bacterial products. In particular, lipopolysaccharide (LPS) from bacterial cell walls binds to CD14 and induces MHC class II molecules and B7. Activated cells also secrete more enzymes, produce more superoxide and reactive nitrogen intermediates and express more Fc and C3b receptors. Receptors for most chemotactic molecules (eg. C5aR) however are downregulated.

COMPLEMENT RECEPTORS

There are four different kinds of receptor (CR1–CR4) for C3b or iC3b, and three of these act as receptors for immune complexes on cells of the mononuclear phagocyte lineage.

CR1 (CD35) is a transmembrane protein consisting of a single polypeptide which occurs on phagocytic cells, where it acts as a receptor for immune complexes. On human erythrocytes it facilitates transport of complexes to phagocytic cells in spleen and liver. On other cells its principal function is to act as a cofactor for factor I. It is also present on some lymphocytes, although its function on these cells is less certain.

CR2 (CD21) is structurally similar to CR1. It forms part of the B cell coreceptor complex and is also present on follicular dendritic cells. It is involved in the uptake of complexes to germinal centres and in the development of B cell memory.

CR3 (CD11b/CD18) is an integrin expressed on mononuclear phagocytes, neutrophils and NK cells, where it facilitates the uptake of immune complexes with bound C3d. It is also involved in monocyte migration into tissues.

CR4 (CD11c/CD18, P150,95) is an integrin which shares a β chain with CR3, and has similar functions, although it is particularly highly expressed on tissue macrophages.

C1q Receptor (C1qR), present on macrophages, binds to the collagenous section of C1q and mannan-binding lectin (MBL) and is thought to be involved in antigen clearance.

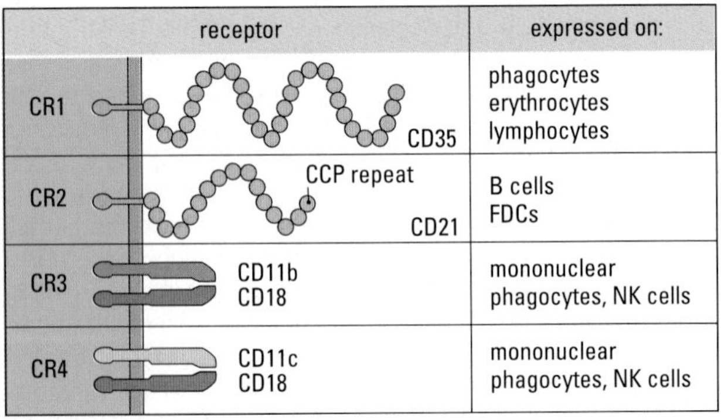

receptor		expressed on:
CR1	CD35	phagocytes erythrocytes lymphocytes
CR2	CCP repeat CD21	B cells FDCs
CR3	CD11b CD18	mononuclear phagocytes, NK cells
CR4	CD11c CD18	mononuclear phagocytes, NK cells

Fig. 3.18 Complement receptors.

Fc RECEPTORS

There are three well-defined receptors for IgG on phagocytic cells which facilitate the uptake of immune complexes, and allow cytotoxic cells to interact with targets. Two receptors for IgE have been described, FcεRI and FcεRII, the first having a role in the control of inflammatory mediator release, the second having an immunoregulatory role.

FcγRI (CD64) is a high-affinity IgG receptor capable of binding monomeric antibody. It is a characteristic marker of mononuclear phagocytes but may also be expressed on activated neutrophils. It is involved in the uptake of immune complexes.

FcγRII (CD32) is a low-affinity receptor present on mononuclear phagocytes, neutrophils, eosinophils, platelets and B cells. On phagocytic cells it appears to facilitate phagocytosis of large complexes, but on B cells it is thought to be involved in control of antibody production. Crosslinking of the surface antibody and Fc receptors on B cells leads to downregulation of the B cell. Activation of platelets by immune complexes bound to their Fc receptors can lead to degranulation, with release of inflammatory mediators.

FcγRIII (CD16) is a low-affinity IgG receptor which occurs in two forms. On NK cells it is a transmembrane glycoprotein (CD16-2) which can crosslink the cells to target cells sensitized with antibody. Engagement of this receptor on NK cells leads to cell activation. On macrophages and neutrophils it is a phosphatidyl-inositol-linked receptor attached to the membrane, where it can bind immune complexes but cannot signal cell activation.

FcεRI is a high-affinity IgE receptor found on mast cells and basophils. These cells can take up monomeric IgE, which sensitizes them. When the particular IgE-binding antigen crosslinks these receptors, it leads to degranulation, with release of histamine and other inflammatory mediators.

FcεRII (CD23) is a low-affinity IgE receptor present on some B cells, with an immunoregulatory function. A soluble form of the receptor acts as a signalling molecule between lymphocytes (see p. 59). It is also present on eosinophils, where it may allow them to engage parasites (eg. schistosomes) coated with IgE.

FcαR (CD89) is expressed on phagocytic cells but also on some B cells and T cells, particularly in Peyer's patches and the lamina propria, hence it is thought to be involved in regulation of IgA synthesis.

CYTOTOXICITY

Cytotoxicity is general term for the ways in which lymphocytes, mononuclear phagocytes and granulocytes can kill target cells. This kind of interaction is important in the destruction of cells which have become infected with viruses, or intracellular microorganisms, which they are unable to eliminate.

T cell-mediated cytotoxicity involves recognition of antigen fragments associated with MHC class I molecules (usually) on the surface of the target cell, and is effected by CD8+ Tc cells. The attacking cell orientates its granules towards the target and releases the contents, including perforin and granzymes, at the junction between the cells. Cytokines such as lymphotoxin or the engagement of CD95 on the target may also signal cell death. The relative contribution of each component depends on the cytotoxic cell type involved. Target cell death occurs by apoptosis.

Fas (CD95) and CD95L. Fas is a molecule belonging to the TNF-R family expressed on many cell types. Ligation of CD95 by its receptor on T cells, CD95L, induces target cell death. Fas has an intracytoplasmic 'death' domain which occurs on other receptors involved in cell survival or death.

Perforin is a pore-forming molecule related to complement C9, which polymerizes on the target cell membrane to form channels.

Granzymes are serine proteases found in the granules of cytotoxic T cells, which may enter target cells via perforin pores to activate enzymes involved in DNA degradation and apoptosis.

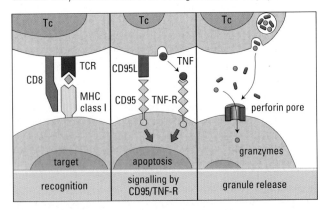

Fig. 3.19 Mechanisms of T cell-mediated cytotoxicity.

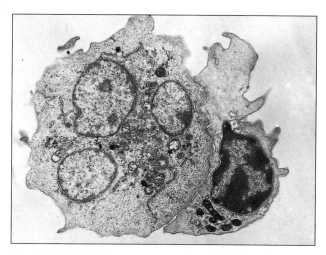

Fig. 3.20 K cell (right) engaging a target cell (left). Courtesy of Mr P. Penfold.

Antibody-Dependent Cell-Mediated Cytotoxicity (ADCC) involves recognition of target cells coated with antibody. This may be effected by LGLs, macrophages or granulocytes, using their Fcγ receptors. The mechanism of cytotoxic damage depends on the effector cell – macrophages can release enzymes and reactive oxygen intermediates, whereas LGLs use perforins and cytokines.

NK cell-mediated cytotoxicity is mediated by LGLs. They kill target cells which fail to express MHC class I molecules or express allogeneic MHC class I. Thus they provide a line of defence against viruses which attempt to evade immune recognition by down-regulating MHC expression. The mechanisms of cytotoxicity are similar to those used by cytotoxic T cells, with granule components (perforin and granzymes) being an important element.

NK cell receptors. Human NK cells are clonally heterogenous and express a variety of receptors that recognize different sets of class I molecules. The receptors develop during NK cell ontogeny so that the ability to recognize self MHC is acquired. One of these receptors, which binds HLA-C, is a two-domain member of the Ig superfamily; another, which recognizes HLA-B and some alleles of HLA-A, is CD94. In mouse, a molecule Ly49, which has a lectin domain, acts as one MHC receptor. Engagement of the MHC receptors inhibits cytotoxicity. NK cells also express activation receptors. These include CD2, CD16 and CD69 in man.

Eosinophil-mediated cytotoxicity. Eosinophils are only weakly phagocytic, and are less efficient than neutrophils and macrophages at destroying endocytosed pathogens. However, they can exocytose their granule contents, releasing factors which are most effective at damaging certain large parasites. Eosinophils recognize targets via bound antibody, including IgE which they bind via FcεRII. Eosinophil degranulation is triggered by ligation of FcεRII or FcγRII. It is also induced *in vitro* by cytokines, including IL-5, TNF, IFN-β and PAF. Eosinophil granule contents include phosphatases, aryl sulphatase and histaminase, in addition to those listed below.

Major Basic Protein (MBP) is a highly cationic protein forming a major component of the crystalloid core of eosinophil granules. It is solubilized before secretion and can damage parasites. Figure 3.21 illustrates progressive damage to schistosomule larvae incubated in MBP.

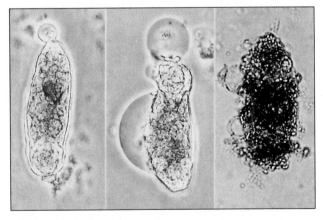

Fig. 3.21 Effect of major basic protein on schistosomule larvae. Courtesy of Dr D. McLaren and Dr Janice Taverne.

Eosinophil Cationic Protein (ECP) is a highly basic, zinc-containing ribonuclease which binds avidly to negatively charged surfaces; it is particularly effective at damaging the tegument of schistosomes.

Eosinophil peroxidase is distinct from myeloperoxidase produced by neutrophils and macrophages, but serves a similar function in the generation of toxic hypohalites.

INFLAMMATION

Inflammation is the response of tissues to injury, with the function of bringing serum molecules and cells of the immune system to the site of damage. The reaction consists of three components:

- Increased blood supply to the region.
- Increased capillary permeability in the affected area.
- Emigration of cells out of the blood vessels and into the tissues.

Inflammation is an ordered process, mediated by the appearance of intercellular adhesion molecules on endothelia and various inflammatory mediators released by tissue cells and leucocytes. Plasma enzyme systems are particularly important sources of inflammatory mediators. These include the complement, clotting, fibrinolytic (plasmin) and kinin systems. Also active are the mediators released by mast cells, basophils and platelets, as well as the eicosanoids generated by many cells at inflammatory sites. Generally, neutrophils are the first cells to appear at acute inflammatory sites, followed by macrophages and lymphocytes, if there is an immunological challenge.

Vasodilation is the dilation of the local blood vessels caused by the actions of mediators such as histamine on the smooth muscle of the vessel wall, allowing increased blood flow.

Transudate/Exudate. Normally, only small molecules pass freely through the capillary wall. The fluid which passes through is a transudate. If inflammation occurs, the endothelial cells are caused to retract, permitting large molecules to pass out as well. This fluid, which is also rich in cells, is an inflammatory exudate.

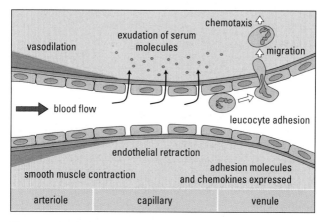

Fig. 3.22 Elements of inflammation.

mediator	origin	actions
histamine	mast cells basophils	increased vascular permeability smooth muscle contraction chemokinesis
5-hydroxy- tryptamine (5HT) = serotonin	platelets mast cells (rodents)	increased vascular permeability smooth muscle contraction
platelet activating factor (PAF)	basophils neutrophils macrophages	mediator release from platelets increased vascular permeability smooth muscle contraction neutrophil activation
neutrophil chemotactic factor (NCF)	mast cells	neutrophil chemotaxis
chemokines	leucocytes	triggering and chemotaxis
C3a	complement C3	mast cell degranulation smooth muscle contraction
C5a	complement C5	mast cell degranulation neutrophil and macrophage chemotaxis, neutrophil activation smooth muscle contraction increased capillary permeability
bradykinin	kinin system (kininogen)	vasodilation smooth muscle contraction increased vascular permeability pain
fibrinopeptides and fibrin break- down products	clotting system	increased vascular permeability neutrophil and macrophage chemotaxis
prostaglandin E2 (PGE2)	cyclooxygenase pathway	vasodilation potentiate increased vascular permeability produced by histamine and bradykinin
leukotriene B4 (LTB4)	lipoxygenase pathway	neutrophil chemotaxis synergizes with PGE2 in increasing vascular permeability
leukotriene D4 (LTD4)	lipoxygenase pathway	smooth muscle contraction increased vascular permeability

Fig. 3.23 Mediators of acute inflammation.

Mediators of inflammation include the plasma enzyme systems, cells of the immune system and products of the pathogens themselves. The principal mediators are listed opposite.

Kinins are generated following tissue injury. Bradykinin is generated by interactions of plasma enzyme systems by the action of kallikrein on high molecular weight kininogen. Lysyl bradykinin (kallidin) is generated by the action of tissue kallikrein on low molecular weight kininogen. They are exceptionally powerful vasoactive mediators.

Eicosanoids are mediators produced from arachidonic acid, which is released from membranes by the action of phospholipase A2. Arachidonic acid is converted into eicosanoids by mast cells and macrophages via two major pathways.

Prostaglandins (PG) and Thromboxanes (Tx) are produced by the action of cyclooxygenase on arachidonic acid. They have diverse proinflammatory effects and often synergize with other mediators.

Leukotrienes (LT) are produced by the lipoxygenase pathway, which generates mediators of acute inflammation and factors important in the later phase of type I hypersensitivity.

Formyl-methionyl (fMet-) peptides (eg. fMLP) are bacterial products which are highly chemotactic for neutrophils.

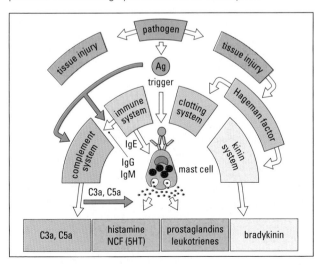

Fig. 3.24 Plasma enzyme systems.

MECHANISMS OF CELL MIGRATION

Leucocyte migration is controlled by molecules expressed on the surface of vascular endothelium that interact with complementary adhesion molecules expressed on different populations of leucocytes. Most leucocyte migration occurs across venules. Several patterns of cell migration can be distinguished, including:

- Movement of lymphocytes into secondary lymphoid tissues.
- Migration of activated lymphocytes to inflammatory sites.
- Migration of neutrophils into tissues during an acute immune response, and migration of mononuclear cells into chronic inflammatory sites.

Each pattern of migration is determined by particular sets of chemokines and adhesion molecules. There are three stages in the adhesion that precedes migration across the endothelium:

1) Slowing and rolling: most leucocyte migration occurs across venules, as the shear force acting on the circulating cells is lower and adhesion molecules are selectively expressed here. Initial slowing is mediated principally by selectins (eg. E-selectin) on the endothelium interacting with carbohydrate on the leucocytes.

2) Triggering: leucocytes may be triggered by chemokines or by the endothelial molecule PECAM (CD31). Chemokines are released at sites of inflammation and may attach to the endothelium to act as flags for the circulating cells. Triggering upregulates the integrins required for firm attachment to the endothelium.

3) Adhesion: the affinity of leucocyte integrins (eg. LFA-1) on activated cells is increased. This allows them to bind to cell adhesion molecules (eg. ICAM-1) induced on the endothelium by inflammatory cytokines. The integrins and the CAMs are attached to the cytoskeleton of either cell and this allows the leucocyte to pull itself across the endothelium. Figure 3.25 shows a lymphocyte adhering to brain endothelium in encephalomyelitis.

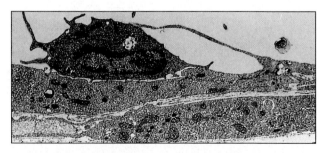

Fig. 3.25 Lymphocyte adhering to CNS endothelium.
Courtesy of Dr Clive Hawkins.

Diapedesis is the process by which cells migrate across the endothelium and into tissues. Adherent cells extend pseudopodia into the junctions between endothelial cells, before squeezing through the gap. In tissues where the endothelia have continuous tight junctions (eg. CNS), migration occurs close to the junctions, but not breaking them apart. Enzymes released by the migrating cells dissolve the basement membrane. New adhesion molecules may now be mobilized to allow the cells to bind cells in the tissue and extracellular matrix components.

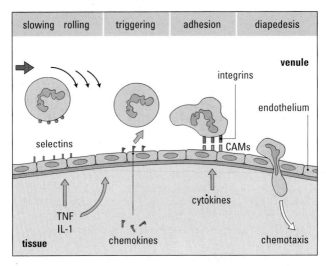

Fig. 3.26 Steps in leucocyte migration into tissues.

Chemotaxis is directional movement of cells in response to an inflammatory mediator. Cells are highly sensitive to, and migrate up, concentration gradients of molecules such as C5a, fMet,Leu,Phe (fMLP) and IL-8; these can all trigger cells on the endothelium.

Chemokinesis is increased random (ie. non-directional) movement of cells caused by inflammatory mediators (eg. histamine).

Adhesion molecules fall into several different structural groups. Some are constitutively expressed by cells (eg. CR3 on mononuclear cells) whereas others may be induced by cytokines or cellular activation. Some adhesion molecules are retained in stores within the cell and may be quickly mobilized to the cell surface (eg. LFA-1 present in neutrophil 'adhesomes'), whereas others (eg. ICAM-1 in endothelium) must be synthesized. The major families of adhesion molecules are listed overleaf:

Selectins are a group of three adhesion molecules with lectin domains that can bind to carbohydrate. P-selectin and E-selectin, induced on endothelium, help to slow migrating leucocytes before adhesion, while L-selectin is expressed on lymphocytes and neutrophils. On lymphocytes it contributes to binding to high endothelial venules in mucosal lymphoid tissues.

PECAM (CD31), expressed on endothelium and some leucocyte populations, can undergo homotypic adhesion, which may activate integrins, or act as a guide during migration.

Integrins consist of an α and β chain, both of which traverse the cell membrane. Usually, the α chain is unique to each molecule, whereas the β chain may be shared with other molecules. Adhesion is dependent on divalent cations — when Mg^{++} is bound, the molecules adopt a high-affinity form. Integrins often have more than one ligand-binding site which recognizes different molecules. Several integrins bind target sequences such as an Arg-Gly-Asp (RGD) sequence in the ligand molecule.

Leucocyte integrins are a family of three molecules which share the β_2 chain (CD18); they include LFA-1 (CD11a/CD18) – important in migration of lymphocytes across endothelium – and CR3 (CD11b/CD18) – expressed on all mononuclear phagocytes – which binds to ICAM-1 on endothelium at sites of inflammation. CR4 (CD11c/CD18) is particularly expressed on tissue macrophages.

VLA (Very Late Antigens) is the designation of the β_1 integrin family, which includes two molecules that appear late on activated T cells and may be involved in binding to extracellular matrix. VLA-4, which binds to VCAM-1, is used by lymphocytes migrating into some inflammatory sites, particularly skin.

CAMs – ICAM-1, ICAM-2, VCAM-1 and MAdCAM-1 belong to the Ig supergene family. ICAM-1 and VCAM-1 are induced on endothelium by IL-1, TNF and IFN-γ, at sites of inflammation; they bind to integrins and mediate adhesion and migration. ICAM-2 is constitutively expressed on endothelium and is thought to control the base level of cell traffic into a tissue. MAdCAM-1, the mucosal addressin, binds both L-selectin and integrins. It controls migration to mucosal lymphoid tissues.

CD44 (Pgp) is a widely distributed molecule also present on leucocytes and thought to be involved in transendothelial migration. It appears to be directed to the leading pseudopod in order to interact with extracellular matrix proteins.

molecule	structure	location	ligand(s)	function
P-selectin	selectin	endothelium neutrophils platelets	sLeX = sialyl Lewis X (carbohydrate)	acute inflammation neutrophil adhesion haemostasis
E-selectin	selectin	endothelium	sialyl Lewis X (eg. CD15)	leucocyte slowing
L-selectin	selectin	lymphocytes neutrophils	sialyl Lewis X	HEV binding slowing
ICAM-1	Ig family	endothelium (inducible)	LFA-1 CR3, CR4	adhesion and migration
ICAM-2	Ig family	endothelium	LFA-1	adhesion and migration
VCAM-1	Ig family	endothelium (inducible)	VLA-4 LPAM	adhesion
MAdCAM-1	Ig family sialylated	lymphoid endothelium	LPAM L-selectin	lymphocyte homing
PECAM	Ig family	endothelium lymphocytes	PECAM ?	adhesion activation migration guidance
LFA-1	$\alpha_L\beta_2$ integrin	leucocytes	ICAM-1, ICAM-2 CR3	migration
CR3	$\alpha_M\beta_2$ integrin	phagocytes	ICAM-1, ICAM-2 C3bi fibronectin	migration immune complex uptake
CR4	$\alpha_X\beta_2$ integrin	phagocytes	ICAM-1 ICAM-2 C3bi	adhesion immune complex uptake
VLA-4	$\alpha_4\beta_1$ integrin	lymphocytes	VCAM-1 LPAM fibronectin	adhesion at inflammatory sites and HEVs
LPAM	$\alpha_4\beta_7$ integrin	lymphocytes	MAdCAM-1	migration to lymphoid tissue
GlyCAM-1	sialoglycoprotein (soluble)	HEV	L-selectin	control of adhesion
PSGL-1	sialoglycoprotein	neutrophils	P-selectin	slowing in acute inflammation
CLA	glycoprotein	lymphocytes	E-selectin	lymphocyte migration to skin

Fig. 3.27 Adhesion molecules involved in leucocyte migration.

COMPLEMENT

Complement is one of the serum enzyme systems. Its functions include mediating inflammation, opsonization of antigenic particles (including microorganisms) and causing membrane damage to pathogens. The system consists of serum molecules, which may be activated via the classical, alternative or lectin pathways. Molecules of the classical pathway are designated C1, C2 etc. Alternative-pathway molecules have letter designations, for example factor B is FB or just B. The properties of the components are given overleaf, and their receptors are on page 68. The complement components interact with each other so that the products of one reaction form the enzyme for the next. Thus, a small initial stimulus can trigger a cascade of activity. Small fragments of complement molecules produced by cleavage are lower case (C3a, C5b). Inactivated enzymes are prefixed 'i' (eg. iC3b), and active enzymes are indicated with a bar (eg. C3b,Bb).

The Classical pathway (backshaded yellow) is activated by immune complexes binding to the C1q subcomponent of C1, which has six Fc binding sites. This causes cleavage of C1r and C1s. C1s then splits C4a from C4, and C2b from C2, leaving C4b,2a, which cleaves C3.

The Alternative pathway (Properdin pathway or Amplification loop) (backshaded purple) is activated in the presence of suitable surfaces or molecules, including microbial products. C3b can bind either H or B. Normally H is bound and C3b is inactivated by I, but in the presence of activators, B is bound and then enzymically cleaved by D, releasing Ba and leaving C3b,Bb, an enzyme that can cleave C3. This gives a feedback amplification loop to generate more C3b.

The Lectin pathway (shaded blue) is activated by MBL binding to bacterial carbohydrates and results in cleavage of C2 and C4.

C3 convertases, including C3b,Bb and C4b,2a, clip C3a from C3 to leave C3b. This has a labile binding site which allows it to bind covalently to nearby molecules with -OH or $-NH_2$ groups. C3b, together with a C3 convertase, can cleave C5.

The Lytic pathway (backshaded orange) is activated when C5b is deposited on membranes. C5b associates with C6, C7, C8 and C9 to form the membrane attack complex.

Membrane attack complex (MAC) is a structure of C5b678 and polymeric C9, which traverses the target cell membrane and allows osmotic leakage from the cell.

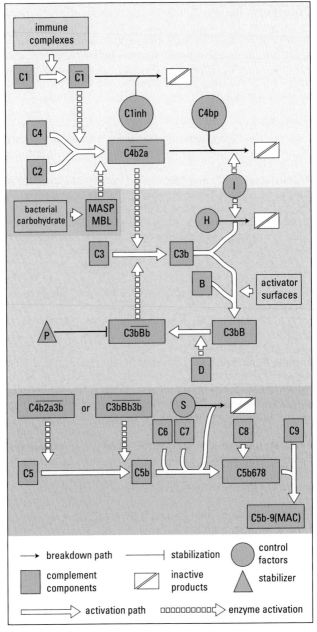

Fig. 3.28 Complement reaction pathways.

Complement fixation is the activation of complement, followed by deposition of the activated components on immune complexes or cell membranes. C3b and C4b can bind covalently to nearby molecules via an internal thioester bond which becomes exposed on activation. The reactive group decays quickly by hydrolysis if a link is not formed. Hence complement is only deposited close to its site of activation.

Bystander lysis is the phenomenon whereby cells in close proximity to a site of complement activation have active components deposited on them and may then be lysed.

Anaphylatoxins C3a and C5a, cleaved from the N-termini of the α chains of C3 and C5, mediate inflammation by causing mast cell degranulation, smooth muscle contraction and increased capillary permeability. C5a is also chemotactic for neutrophils and monocytes. In this way these peptides mimic some of the reactions of anaphylaxis. They are substantially inactivated by removal of their C-terminal Arg residue by serum carboxypeptidases.

Collectins – Mannan-Binding Lectin (MBL) and conglutinin. The collectins are a group of carbohydrate-binding polymeric proteins which include MBL and conglutinin (structurally related to C1q). Both can initiate complement activation.

Control of complement activation is effected by the natural decay of the enzymically active convertases and the actions of the various inhibitors and inactivators listed opposite. Membrane-associated molecules also alter the rate of complement breakdown. In particular, CR1, FH and DAF promote the decay of C3b,Bb.

Decay-Accelerating Factor (DAF, CD55) and Membrane Cofactor Protein (MCP, CD46) are proteins normally present on many mammalian cell membranes which limit the activity of the alternative pathway and the development of C5 convertases.

Homologous Restriction Factors (HRF & CD59) are membrane proteins which limit the activity of autologous C8 and C9.

Paroxysmal nocturnal haemoglobinuria is a condition in which red cell breakdown occurs via the alternative pathway. Patients' red cells are deficient in control proteins (particularly DAF).

Hereditary angioedema is due to a genetic deficiency of C1inh. There is uncontrolled local activation of C2, which undergoes conversion into a kinin that induces pathological local oedema.

component	mol. wt (kD)	serum conc. (μg/ml)	no. of poly-peptides	function
C1q	410	150	18	form a Ca^{++}-linked complex – C1q
C1r	83	50	1	C1r$_2$ C1s$_2$; C1q binds to complexed Ig
C1s	83	50	1	to activate the classical pathway
C4	210	550	3	classical pathway molecules, activated by C1s to form a C3
C2	115	25	1	convertase, C4b,2a
C3	180	1200	2	active C3 (C3b) opsonizes anything to which it binds and activates the lytic pathway. C3a causes mast cell degranulation and smooth muscle contraction. iC3b, C3d, C3e and C3g are breakdown products of C3b
C5	180	70	2	C5b on membranes initiates the lytic pathway. C5a is chemotactic for macrophages and neutrophils, causes smooth muscle contraction, mast cell degranulation and increased capillary permeability
C6	130	60	1	lytic pathway components which
C7	120	50	1	assemble in the presence of C5b to
C8	155	55	3	form the membrane attack complex
C9	75	60	1	and so may cause cell lysis
B	95	200	1	B binds to C3b in the presence of alternative pathway activators, then is
D	25	10	1	cleaved by D, an active serum enzyme, to form a C3 convertase C3b,Bb
P (properdin)	185	25	4	stabilizes C3b,Bb to potentiate amplification loop activity
MBL	540	1	18	binds bacterial carbohydrate
MASP	94	?	1	activates C4 and C2
C4bp	550	250	7	C4bp binds C4b, and H binds C3b
H(β_1H)	150	500	1	to act as cofactors for I, which cleaves
I(C3bina)	100	30	2	and inactivates C3b and C4b
C1inh	100	185	1	binds and inactivates C$\overline{1r}_2$ and C$\overline{1s}_2$
S-protein (vitro-nectin)	83	505	1	binds C5b-7, prevents attachment to membranes

Fig. 3.29 The complement components.

IMMUNOREGULATION

The immune response is regulated primarily by antigen, and secondarily by interactions between lymphocytes, APCs and their products, including antibody and cytokines. Antigen is the primary initiator of immune responses, since the first signal required to trigger lymphocytes is antigen or antigen/MHC. Indeed, the immune system may be viewed as a single homeostatic unit for the elimination of antigen. In this view, antigen initiates an immune response that eliminates that antigen, and the immune system then returns to the resting state. The essential role of antigen is seen at the cellular level. For example, antigen/MHC triggers T cell activation, and expression of receptors for cytokines (eg. IL-2) required for T cell division. T cell help causes B cells to produce specific antibody, leading to elimination of the antigen. With the disappearance of antigen, there is no longer any first activation signal for the B cells. Likewise, the lack of an antigen/MHC activation signal for the T cells causes them to lose their cytokine receptors and stop cytokine production. The immune system then falls back to the resting state.

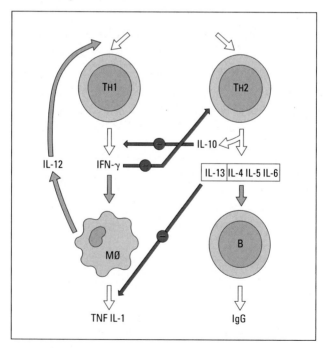

Fig. 3.30 Immunoregulation: TH1-and TH2-type responses.

Antibody-mediated immunoregulation. Antibody regulates its own production in several ways: 1) Binding to antigen, so preventing it from activating lymphocytes; 2) Binding to Fc receptors on B cells, which in the presence of antigen causes crosslinking of the Fc receptors and surface Ig. This delivers an inhibitory signal to the cells; 3) Promoting immune complex formation and localization of antigen to germinal centres, so promoting Ig class switching and induction of B cell memory.

Network hypothesis is a theory that lymphocytes may be regulated in their interactions by recognition of the idiotypes on the antigen receptors of other cells, or by idiotype-bearing antibodies. For example, an anti-idiotypic antibody could cause the downregulation of the set of B cells expressing the idiotype. The theory does not make predictions as to whether the interactions will be enhancing or suppressive. Such regulation is secondary to that mediated by antigen and cytokines because of the enormous redundancy in the immune system – if clones of cells are downregulated, their functions are usually taken by other clones.

Suppression. A regulatory group of T cells (T suppressors, Ts) modulate the activity of other lymphocytes. Early experiments indicated that Ts cells were CD8+, but no specific marker for these cells has been identified and CD4+ cells can also sometimes be suppressive. This is, therefore, a functional definition. Suppression is an active process and can be distinguished from tolerance by transferring the suppression with T cells. The cellular basis for this type of immunoregulation involves some or all of the following mechanisms: 1) A specific cytostatic action of CD8+ Tc cells; 2) Passive blocking of lymphocyte activation by sequestering essential cytokines required for cell division; 3) Secretion of immunosuppressive molecules such as prostaglandins or TGF-β; 4) An immunoregulatory effect caused by the local production of specific sets of cytokines, causing cells to switch between different modes of immune response (see below); 5) Induction of clonal anergy due to the Ts cells supplying an activation signal but not the required costimulatory signals or cytokines.

TH1- and TH2-type responses. The TH1 subset promotes cell-mediated immune responses, while TH2 promotes antibody-mediated responses, including IgE production (see opposite). Moreover, each mode of response suppresses the other. IFN-γ produced by TH1 cells limits proliferation of TH2 cells, while IL-12 from mononuclear phagocytes promotes development of TH1 cells. Conversely, IL-10 from TH2 cells prevents cytokine production by TH1 cells, and IL-13 inhibits macrophage cytokine production.

NEUROENDOCRINE REGULATION OF IMMUNE RESPONSES

There is evidence that neurological events can affect immunological functions, either directly or via the endocrine system.

Innervation of lymphoid tissues. Thymus, spleen and lymph nodes all receive sympathetic noradrenergic innervation. They control blood flow through the lymphoid tissues, thus affecting lymphocyte traffic. However, fibres also run between the lymphocytes and appear to form junctions with individual cells. Denervation of lymphoid tissues can modulate immune responses.

Pituitary/adrenal axis. Stress can induce release of adrenocorticotrophic hormone (ACTH) from the pituitary. This induces release of glucocorticoids, which are immunosuppressive. Lymphocytes also produce ACTH in response to corticotrophin-releasing factor In addition, the adrenal medulla releases catecholamines which can alter leucocyte migration patterns and lymphocyte responsiveness.

Endocrine and neuropeptide regulation. Lymphocytes carry receptors for many hormones, including insulin, thyroxine, growth hormone and somatostatin. These hormones, as well as enkephalins and endorphins released during stress, modulate T and B cell functions in complex ways, depending on the level of mediators.

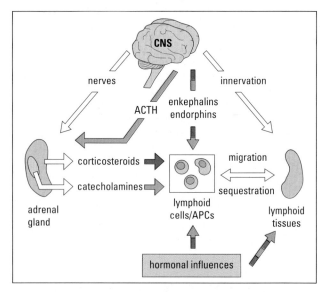

Fig. 3.31 Neuroendocrine regulation of immune responses.

IMMUNE RESPONSE GENES

Responder and Non-responder strains. Inbred strains of animals produce a characteristic level of immune response to injected antigens. The status depends mostly on MHC-linked immune response genes and varies with different antigens. Genes of the *TCR* loci and *IG* loci also affect responses to particular antigens. Loci which control antigen processing and cytokine production contribute to the overall control of responses.

MHC-linked Ir genes. The most important Ir genes encode class II MHC molecules, which control the way in which each antigen is presented. There is also some haplotypic variation in genes controlling antigen processing (DM, TAP etc.).

Repertoire is the sum total of antigen receptors produced by the immune system. The initial repertoire is partly determined by the genes of the TCR and antibody H and L chains.

Clonal restriction. This refers to an immune response produced by a limited number of clones. For example, the primary immune response to phosphoryl choline in Ig^a haplotype mice is predominantly generated by B cells expressing the T15 idiotype. T cell responses can also be clonally restricted with selective use of particular T cell receptor V genes. This is related to selective antigen presentation by particular MHC molecules.

Biozzi mice are strains genetically inbred to give high or low antibody responses to an antigen (originally sheep erythrocytes). At least 10 separate non-MHC gene loci control responsiveness in these animals. The high- and low-responder strains differ in the way their macrophages handle antigens – low responders degrade antigen quickly and do not present it.

macrophage function	low responder	high responder
1. antigen uptake	+ + +	+
2. lysosomal enzyme activity	+ + +	+
3. intracellular degradation of antigen	+ + +	+
4. surface persistence of antigen	+	+ + +

Fig. 3.32 Macrophage functions in Biozzi mice.

IMMUNOSUPPRESSION

Immunosuppression describes measures used to reduce immune responses, particularly in transplantation surgery (to prevent graft rejection) and in the control of autoimmune diseases. Most measures are not antigen specific, although some drugs have greater effects on the immune system than other tissues.

Steroids, including glucocorticosteroids, corticosteroids and synthetic steroids such as dexamethasone, have numerous immunosuppressive and anti-inflammatory effects, macrophages being particularly sensitive. They inhibit arachidonic acid release and hence reduce eicosanoid production. They also reduce secretion of neutral proteases and IL-1. Steroids interfere with antigen presentation, inhibit the primary antibody response and reduce the numbers of circulating T cells.

Azathioprine and 6-Mercaptopurine are purine analogues which act on small lymphocytes and dividing cells, thereby blocking development of effector cells. Monocytes are reduced, and K cell activity is also inhibited.

Cyclophosphamide and Chlorambucil are alkylating agents which damage DNA and prevent its replication. They act primarily on lymphocytes and strongly inhibit antibody responses, but have little effect on phagocytes. Experimentally, cyclophosphamide prevents B cells from regenerating their receptors.

Cyclosporin-A is a fungal metabolite which interferes with cytokine production by T cells, particularly IL-2, and inhibits IL-2R expression – early events in lymphocyte activation. It does not affect lymphoblasts, nor is it anti-mitotic or cytotoxic. It is the drug of first choice in transplantation surgery.

Fk506 is a bacterial compound which prevents T cell activation by inhibiting the action of calcineurin, an enzyme required for transduction of signals from the T cell receptor.

Rapamycin inhibits the ability of T cell growth factors to put T cells into cell cycle. Both rapamycin and Fk506 bind to the same receptor, although their modes of action are different.

Antagonist peptides are analogues of peptides which bind to MHC molecules of particular haplotypes. Such peptides are an experimental treatment for autoimmune conditions. By occupying the MHC-binding site, they block access for autoantigen peptides.

IMMUNOPOTENTIATION

Biological Response Modifiers (BRMs) are compounds which modify an immune response, usually enhancing it. They include immunopotentiating bacterial products, chemicals such as polynucleotides and physiologically active molecules including cytokines, as well as the true adjuvants which are administered together with antigen. A number of these substances have been used in an attempt to potentiate immune reactions in cancer patients and immunodeficiency. Many of the bacterial products act by inducing cytokine production or the expression of costimulatory molecules on antigen-presenting cells. Bacterial products include:

BCG (Bacillus Calmette-Guerin) is a live non-virulent strain of *Mycobacterium bovis* which is used in vaccines for immunization against tuberculosis.

Muramyl dipeptide (MDP) is the smallest adjuvant active part of BCG extractable from the cell wall.

Corynebacterium parvum induces lymphoid hyperplasia and activates macrophages.

Bordetella pertussis produces a lymphocytosis-promoting factor (LPF) which is a T cell mitogen and an immunostimulant. *B. pertussis* causes whooping cough.

Endotoxin/Lipopolysaccharide (LPS) is a component of Gram-negative bacterial cell walls. It is mitogenic for B cells and activates macrophages following binding to its receptor CD14.

Adjuvants are compounds which enhance the immune response when administered with antigen, thereby producing higher antibody titres and prolonged production. The distinction between primary and secondary immune responses becomes blurred when adjuvants are used.

Thymic hormones are factors produced by the thymus, which assist T cell development in the thymus and their maintenance in the periphery. They include thymosin, thymopoietin, thymostimulin and Facteur Thymique Serique (FTS).

Lymphokine-Activated Killer (LAK) cells are syngeneic cytotoxic T cells generated *in vitro* by treating an individual's cells with cytokines, such as IL-2 and IFN-γ. They are sometimes reinfused into patients for cancer immunotherapy.

TOLERANCE

Tolerance is the acquisition of non-responsiveness to a molecule recognized by the immune system. Whether a molecule induces an immune response or tolerance is largely determined by the way in which it is first presented to the immune system.

Neonatal tolerance. Neonatal animals are very susceptible to the induction of tolerance because of the general immaturity of their immune systems. Consequently, tolerance induced at this stage of life is very persistent.

Self tolerance. It is observed that animals generally tolerate their own tissues – if they do not, autoimmune disease may result. Self tolerance is thought to be due primarily to clonal deletion of cells in the neonatal period. As new mature lymphocytes develop, they too are aborted just when they are most susceptible to tolerization.

Central tolerance refers to the induction of tolerance during lymphocyte development. Self-reactive T cells are deleted in the thymus and self-reactive B cells in the bone marrow.

Peripheral tolerance is a necessary mechanism for maintaining tolerance to antigens which are not present in the primary lymphoid organs, or where the receptor is of low affinity.

B cell tolerance. In general, immature cells are more susceptible to tolerance induction than mature cells, and can be tolerized by smaller doses of tolerogens. The dose of antigen and the way it is presented are critical. Self-reactive B cells fail to express Bcl-2 during development in the bone or secondary lymphoid tissues and thus die by apoptosis. In the bone marrow, autoreactive B cells may escape deletion by editing their receptor specificity – making a new light-chain rearrangement. B cells may also become anergic to their antigen if they receive incomplete activation signals. Such cells downregulate surface IgM while retaining IgD.

T cell tolerance. T cells are more easily tolerized than B cells. Once established, the duration of T cell tolerance in an animal is usually longer than that of the B cells. Immature T cells may be deleted during thymic development, although cells with low-avidity receptors remain. Mature T cells can be made anergic depending on how the antigen is presented to them. In particular, lack of suitable costimulatory signals by APCs can induce tolerance. Since B cells require help from T_H2 cells, B cell tolerance may be consequent on T cell tolerance.

Superantigens are antigens which associate particularly effectively with MHC molecules and can induce clonal deletion of T cells that recognize them. Potentially, they can modulate the repertoire of T cells generated.

High-zone and Low-zone tolerance. Tolerance is best induced by high levels of antigen (high zone), which tolerizes B cells. However, some antigens in subimmunogenic doses (low zone) can also tolerize the T cell populations.

Enhancement includes ways of inducing tolerance in transplantation surgery, which enhances graft survival. The mechanism often involves interference with antigen presentation, for example by administration of anti-MHC class II antibody to block T cell-mediated recognition of graft.

Tolerance mechanisms. Several mechanisms maintain tolerance to self tissues (Fig. 3.33):
- Sequestration of antigen away from the immune system.
- Central or peripheral tolerance induction of B cells and T cells.
- Failure to process and present autoantigens by APCs.
- Absence of costimulatory molecules on APCs.
- Suppressive cytokines, including IL-10 and TGF-β.

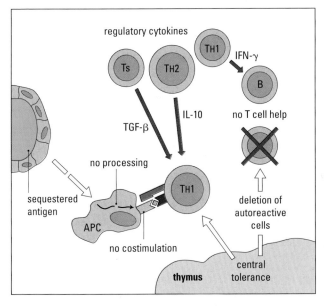

Fig. 3.33 Mechanisms for maintenance of self tolerance.

Immunopathology | 4

IMMUNODEFICIENCY

Immunodeficiency is often identified in individuals by their increased susceptibility to infection, caused by a failure of one or more divisions of the immune system. Primary immunodeficiencies are inherited and may affect any part of the system. Examples include failure of lymphocyte development, impaired granulocyte functions, lack of macrophage receptors and absence of particular complement components. These deficiencies usually become apparent in the early months of life as immunity conferred by maternal antibodies wanes. Secondary, or acquired, immunodeficiency is a consequence of many pathogenic infections, some of which directly attack the immune system (eg. HIV infection), while others (eg. malaria) subvert effective immune responses.

Severe Combined Immunodeficiency (SCID) is a group of conditions with leucopenia, impaired cell-mediated immunity, low or absent antibody levels and undeveloped secondary lymphoid tissues. Some cases can be attributed to autosomal recessive adenosine deaminase deficiency or purine nucleoside phosphorylase deficiency. Other cases in which these enzymes are unaffected

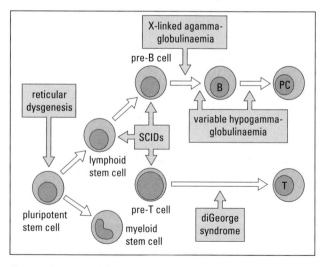

Fig. 4.1 Immunodeficiencies.

may be X-linked or autosomal recessive traits, and one type is due to inability to recombine antigen receptor molecules. The different forms of SCID may be correlated with the points on the lymphomyeloid differentiation pathways at which the deficiencies act.

DiGeorge and Nezelof syndromes, due to failed development of the third and fourth pharyngeal pouches, result in thymic hypoplasia with low numbers of functionally active T cells. T cell numbers may rise to normal within 1–2 years.

X-linked agammaglobulinaemia (Bruton's disease). Patients with this condition have normal T cell functions and cell-mediated immunity to viral infections, but have very low immunoglobulin levels and cannot make antibody responses. The B cells fail to express a tyrosine kinase btk required for the maturation of pre-B cells into mature B cells.

X-linked hyper-IgM (HIGM) is principally due to mutation in CD40L, the T cell ligand which binds to CD40 on B cells – an interaction required for class switching in secondary responses.

Common Variable Immunodeficiency (CVID) is a variety of conditions with no clear pattern of inheritance, which affect B cell differentiation – B cells are often present, but do not develop into plasma cells because of lack of T cell help. There is a relatively high incidence of autoimmunity and lymphoreticular neoplasias.

Ataxia telangiectasia, a neurological disease, also has an associated immunodeficiency. There is reduced T cell function, and some Ig subclasses are deficient. It is caused by an inability to repair DNA, and chromosomal breaks occur in the Ig genes.

Wiskott Aldrich syndrome has a severe associated immunodeficiency in which T cells make ineffective responses to antigens. Lymphocyte numbers are near normal, but antibody subclasses are abnormal and antibody is rapidly catabolized.

Thymoma, a thymocyte neoplasia, is associated with immunodeficiency and a number of autoimmune diseases, including myasthenia gravis and haemolytic anaemia.

MHC class II deficiency (Bare leucocyte syndrome) is caused by a lack of promotors which bind to the 5' controlling regions of the MHC class II genes. The absence of class II causes impaired T cell education in the thymus. Patients have recurrent infections, particularly of the gastrointestinal tract.

Acquired Immune Deficiency Syndrome (AIDS) is due to infection with the retroviruses HIV-1 or HIV-2, which infect cells expressing CD4, including T helper cells and some APCs. Following infection, some individuals have a transient fever. This may develop into a generalized lymphadenopathy. Gradually, CD4+ T cell deficiency develops and this is associated with opportunistic infections and sometimes a fast-growing form of Kaposi's sarcoma. B cells, Tc cells and phagocytes may be affected secondarily.

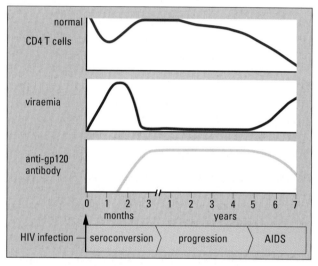

Fig. 4.2 Serology of HIV infection.

Chronic Granulomatous Disease (CGD) is due to a defect in NADPH oxidase, resulting in impaired oxygen-dependent killing by macrophages. Infection with pyogenic bacteria (particularly those producing catalase) occurs and macrophages accumulate at sites of chronic inflammation, forming granulomas.

Chediak Higashi syndrome is a condition with impaired phagocyte responses to chemoattractants and reduced killing of phagocytosed bacteria. A cytoskeletal defect underlies the condition.

Leucocyte adhesion deficiency (Lad-1, Lad-2) is characterized by impaired neutrophil localization to tissues and impaired phagocytosis. Lad-1 is due to lack of CD18, the common β chain of the integrins LFA-1, CR3 and CR4, used in cell migration and phagocytosis. Lad-2 is due to defective glycosylation, resulting in lack of ligands for E-selectin and P-selectin, needed for migration.

MHC TYPING

MHC nomenclature. MHC molecules are highly polymorphic, varying between individuals and loci. Take, for example, the variant DRB1*0406. This is a variant of the HLA-DR region at the B1 region which encodes the first of the DR-β chains. The variant produces a molecule with the specificity DR4 (04) and is the sixth genetic variant discovered at the locus that produces this specificity (06).

Tissue typing is the technique used to determine the MHC speci-ficities carried on an individual's cells. Typing is performed by adding antisera of defined specificity (eg. anti-HLA-DR4) to the cell to be typed (usually lymphocytes). Addition of complement kills the cells, which can be visualized by staining with (eg.) trypan blue.

Typing sera specific for particular MHC molecules were originally made by immunizing allogeneic individuals with cells and absorb-ing out unwanted specificities. This has largely been superseded by haplotype-specific monoclonal antibodies.

Public (Supratypic) and Private specificities. Antibodies raised against framework parts of MHC molecules often cross-react with several MHC antigens; these recognize public specificities. In contrast, antibodies which bind to only one MHC molecule are said to recognize private specificities.

Mixed Lymphocyte Culture/Reaction (MLC/MLR) is a tech-nique for typing cells, in which lymphocytes of different individuals are cocultured. If the cells differ, they are stimulated to divide. The test can be performed either with each set of cells reacting to the other (two-way MLR), or with one set (stimulator) treated so that it cannot respond and only the proliferation of the responding (test) cells is measured (one-way MLR). A lack of response indicates that the test cell and typing cell share an MHC specificity.

Homozygous typing cells, used in MLC, are cells with two identical MHC haplotypes. Human typing cells often come from the offspring of first-cousin marriages.

Primed Lymphocyte Test (PLT). This is a highly sensitive MLC assay for detecting determinants which stimulate allogeneic T cells. The test cells are mixed with lymphocytes previously primed to a particular determinant by coculture with homozygous typing cells. In a subsequent coculture, the primed cells proliferate rapidly if the test cell carries the same determinant as the original homozygous priming cell – primed cells, not the test cells, proliferate.

TRANSPLANTATION

Grafts will be accepted if the recipient shares histocompatibility genes with the graft donor. So, for example, a strain A mouse accepts a strain A graft but not a strain B graft. The $(A \times B)F_1$ mouse accepts the B graft because it has B genes, but the B mouse rejects the $(A \times B)F_1$ graft because it lacks the A genes.

Histocompatibility genes determine whether a graft is accepted. A large number of gene loci affect rejection, but the MHC is most important. Although the MHC was first identified for its role in graft rejection, this is not its physiological function.

Minor histocompatibility loci encode allelically variable molecules which induce weak graft rejection. Such molecules are processed and presented by the MHC class I molecules of the graft cells. In man, even in MHC-matched transplants (eg. between siblings), graft rejection reactions can still occur because of minor-locus differences. Reactions induced by these antigens can usually be suppressed, whereas reactions due to major-locus (MHC) differences cannot.

Passenger cells are donor leucocytes present in graft tissue. They are particularly important in sensitizing recipient TH cells to donor antigens, since they express MHC class II molecules and can migrate into the host lymphatic system.

First and Second set rejection. The immune reactions which produce graft rejection display specificity and memory. For example, a skin allograft in man will normally be rejected in 10–14 days, but if a second allograft with the same tissue type is given the recipient will reject it more rapidly, usually in 5–7 days.

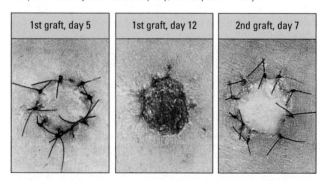

| 1st graft, day 5 | 1st graft, day 12 | 2nd graft, day 7 |

Fig. 4.3 Graft rejection displays immunological memory.

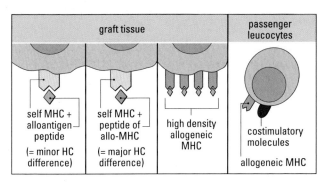

Fig. 4.4 Ways in which graft alloantigens may be presented.

Crossmatching. To avoid graft rejection, the tissue type of the donor and recipient are crossmatched. All donor/recipient pairs are matched for the ABO blood group, and for as many class I and II specificities as possible. The greater the number of shared specificities (particularly class II), the higher the chance of graft survival.

Rejection reactions are induced by recipient TH cells which recognize allogeneic MHC molecules. These activate graft-infiltrating mononuclear cells to damage the graft. Alternatively, Tc cells recognizing allogeneic class I MHC molecules can kill them.

Privileged tissues and sites. Some allogeneic graft tissues (eg. liver) induce only weak immune reactions. One explanation is that the privileged tissues express relatively few MHC antigens. Privileged sites are areas where grafts are mostly isolated from the immune system; eg. the cornea lacks a lymphatic drainage.

Hyperacute/Acute/Chronic rejection describe the speed of rejection in organs such as the kidney. Hyperacute reactions occur within minutes of implantation and are caused by preformed antibody to the graft. Acute rejection occurs within two weeks of grafting and is due to prior sensitization of the recipient to histocompatibility antigens. Chronic rejection develops later and is due to the development of sensitivity to graft antigens. This sometimes occurs after the cessation of immunosuppression, necessitated by infection.

Graft versus Host Disease (GvHD) may occur when immunocompetent donor cells (eg. from a bone marrow graft) recognize and react against the recipient's tissues, because the recipient is either immunosuppressed or cannot recognize the allogeneic cells. Sensitized donor TH cells recruit macrophages, to cause pathological damage, especially in skin, gut epithelium and liver.

MHC DISEASE ASSOCIATIONS

Virtually every disease involving immune reactions is preferentially associated with particular haplotypes of MHC molecules. For example, individuals with the class I molecule HLA-B27 are 90 times more likely to develop ankylosing spondylitis than people lacking this allele. The table opposite lists some of the diseases which show strong associations with particular MHC haplotypes. These disease associations are due to two factors that are central to the workings of the immune system: 1) MHC molecules are highly polymorphic, ie. varying between loci and between individuals; 2) MHC molecules are central to all aspects of antigen presentation. The corollary is that different MHC molecules may be better or worse at presenting different antigen peptides to T cells – some haplotypes permit strong immune responses, whereas others only allow weak ones. Indeed, MHC class II molecules were first identified as immune response (Ir) genes. It follows that, as MHC genes control the ability to make immune responses, they also partly control disease susceptibility in any condition where immune reactions occur.

Relative risk is the risk of developing a disease when a particular HLA haplotype is present compared with when it is absent. A relative risk of greater than one indicates that the haplotype is more prevalent in patients than in normal individuals, whereas a relative risk of less than one indicates a protective effect.

Linkage occurs between sets of genes on a single chromosome, such as the HLA complex. Unless crossover between maternal and paternal chromosomes occurs, a linked gene complex will be inherited as a block. Some diseases such as narcolepsy show strong MHC association due to their real disease-susceptibility gene being in strong linkage disequilibrium with the DR2 haplotype.

Linkage disequilibrium refers to the finding that some pairs of genes are found together more frequently than would be expected by chance – ie. more than the product of their individual gene frequencies. There are two possible explanations for this: 1) There is a selective advantage in inheriting the entire block of genes; 2) Two genes have appeared together by chance, and there has been insufficient evolutionary time to separate them. Many sets of MHC molecules are linked, eg. HLA-A1 with HLA-B8, and HLA-A3 with HLA-B7. Consequently, if one MHC molecule is associated with a disease, any linked haplotypes will also be associated with the disease, although they do not necessarily contribute to the disease association.

disease	specificity	relative risk*
rheumatoid arthritis	DR4	5.8
	DR3	5.0
	DR3 and DR4	14.0
juvenile rheumatoid arthritis	B27	4.5
	Dw14	47.0
	Dw4	26.0
ankylosing spondylitis	B27	87.0
Reiter's disease	B27	33.0
post-shigella arthritis	B27	20.7
post-salmonella arthritis	B27	17.6
Graves' disease	DR3	3.5
	B35	5.0
Hashimoto's thyroiditis	DR3	2.6
Addison's disease	DR3	8.8
insulin-dependent diabetes	DR3	5.7
	DR4	6.4
	DR2	0.2
multiple sclerosis	DR2	3.8
myasthenia gravis	B8	3.4
psoriasis vulgaris	B37	6.4
	B13	4.7
	B17	4.7
	Cw6	13.3
dermatitis herpetiformis	B8	8.7
	DR3	56.4
Goodpasture's syndrome	DR2	13.1
chronic active hepatitis	B8	9.0
	DR3	13.9
coeliac disease	B8	8.3
	DR3	10.9
haemochromatosis	A3	8.2
	B14	4.7

Fig. 4.5 MHC disease associations (European caucasoids).
*Precise values vary between studies.

AUTOIMMUNE DISEASE

Autoantigens/Autoantibodies refer to self molecules recognized as antigens and the antibodies which react against them.

Autoreactive cells are lymphocytes with receptors for autoantigens. These cells can potentially produce an autoimmune response but do not necessarily do so.

Autoimmunity is the reaction of the immune system against the body's own tissues. To understand how autoimmune reactions can develop it is necessary to know the mechanisms by which self tolerance is normally maintained. These include: 1) Sequestration of autoantigen; 2) Deletion of autoreactive lymphocytes in thymus or bone marrow; 3) Failure to process and present particular self molecules; 4) Induction of anergy in autoreactive T cells, because of lack of costimulatory signals; 5) Suppressive cytokines and hormones (see p. 91).

T cell bypass. Most self-reactive T cells are deleted or anergized, but autoreactive B cells may become activated by a mechanism which bypasses the tolerant T cells. For example, a cross-reactive exogenous antigen taken up by an autoreactive B cell could be presented to a T cell recognizing a non-self epitope, which then helps the B cell (Fig. 4.6a). Alternatively, polyclonal stimulators such as Epstein-Barr virus could stimulate the B cells directly.

T cell autoreactivity may also be induced by cross-reactive microbial antigens. In Fig. 4.6b, microbial adjuvants (eg. LPS) induce costimulatory molecules on the macrophage, activating a quiescent autoreactive T cell. In Fig. 4.6c, an enveloped virus is internalized by a macrophage and processed in the class II pathway. The viral envelope contains self molecules which are now presented. In Fig. 4.6d, a quiescent self-reactive T cell is stimulated by a cross-reactive microbial antigen. After priming, the T cell expresses new costimulatory molecules and is more readily activated if presented with self antigen.

Autoregulatory failure. A breakdown in central or peripheral tolerance may produce autoimmunity (Fig. 4.6e).

Organ-specific autoimmune diseases are directed primarily at particular tissues, eg. anti-thyroglobulin in Hashimoto's thyroiditis or to pancreatic β cells in diabetes. Organ-specific autoantibodies tend to occur together in particular individuals and their relatives.

Organ non-specific autoimmune diseases are directed to widely distributed autoantigens, such as the anti-DNA antibody in systemic lupus erythematosus. These conditions often produce type III immune complex-mediated hypersensitivity reactions.

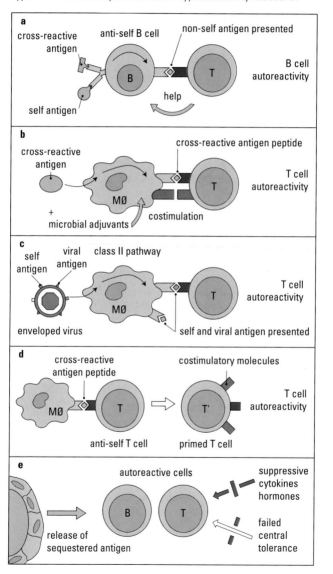

Fig. 4.6 Mechanisms for breakdown of self tolerance.

ANIMAL MODELS AND MUTANT STRAINS

Different strains of animals with impaired immune systems have been particularly useful in modelling human immunodeficiencies and autoimmune diseases. It must be emphasized that the resemblance may only be in the appearance of the diseases. In some cases (eg. nude strains) the defect is determined by a single gene locus, but autoimmunity in the autoimmune strains depends on multiple genetic loci, which interact with each other. Figure 4.7 lists some of the more important strains.

Inbred strains of animals are made by repeated brother × sister matings in successive generations, giving a strain with identical sets of autosomes. If by chance a pair of identical chromosomes occurs in the F_1 animals, inbreeding ensures that the pair remains fixed in the genome of subsequent generations. By repeated inbreeding, all the chromosome pairs become (and will remain) homozygous.

Recombinant strains are produced by crossing different inbred strains. On rare occasions, crossing over occurs in the F_1 animal so that the affected chromosome has different haplotypes at each end. These strains are used to identify the segment of chromosome responsible for a particular characteristic.

Recombinant inbred strains are produced by crossing strains (a × b) and then inbreeding from the offspring. This gives strains which have identical sets of chromosomes, but each set will either be of the a type or b type at random. They are used to determine which chromosomes carry the genes for each trait.

Congenic strains are bred to be identical to each other except at some chosen locus. For example, an H-2^k congenic animal would have the MHC locus of the k haplotype superimposed on a background of genes from a non-H-2^k strain.

bm mutants are strains of mice derived from an H-2^b strain which developed mutations in the H-2 region. Mice with these mutations, designated H2^{bm}, induce graft rejection reactions in H-2^b mice.

Transgenic strains are derived from a founder animal which has had new/variant genes inserted at the fertilized-embryo stage. All cells of a transgenic animal carry the new genes, although they may only be expressed in some cell lineages.

Knockout strains are transgenic animals with targeted deletions or mutations of specific genes.

strain/species	characteristics
nude mouse, nude rat	The nude mutants (nu) lack a thymus and all T cells A linked locus produces hairlessness
beige mouse (Bg)	NK cell and granulocyte defects affecting degranulation, elastase and cathepsin G
NZB mouse	Autoimmunity with haemolytic anaemia and impaired immunoregulation (polygenic)
(NZB × NZW) F$_1$	Autoimmunity with immune complex nephritis, used as SLE model (polygenic)
MRL.lpr or gld mouse	T cell lymphoproliferation The lpr mutation affects CD95 (fas), and the gld mutation, CD95L
Nod mouse (non-obese diabetic)	Autoimmune reaction to pancreatic β cells Model of type II diabetes (polygenic)
BXSB mouse	Y-chromosome linked Yaa mutation accelerates autoimmunity
SCID mouse	Fails to recombine Ig or TCR genes due to defect in DNA repair enzyme, DNA-PKcs
CBA/N mouse	Lacks CD5 B cell subset X-linked deficiency (Xid) in a kinase (btk) required in Ig and CD40 signalling
C3H/HeJ mouse	B cells lack receptor for LPS
DBA/2	Impaired B cell development Mutation in kinase domain of cKit
motheaten (mev) mouse	Severe B cell deficiency Lacks a protein tyrosine phosphatase (PTP1c)
B/B rat	Spontaneous autoimmune diabetes and thyroid autoimmunity
buffalo rat	A proportion develop autoimmune thyroiditis and/or diabetes
obese chicken	Autoimmune thyroiditis – model of Hashimoto's disease

Fig. 4.7 Characteristics of immunologically aberrant strains.

HYPERSENSITIVITY

Hypersensitivity describes an immune response which occurs in an exaggerated or inappropriate form. In some cases responses may occur against innocuous external antigens, such as pollen in hayfever. In other cases responses against genuine pathogens are generated which are out of proportion to the damage caused by the pathogen. Also of great importance are the different kinds of tissue damage seen in autoimmune diseases: these are in effect hypersensitivity reactions, since any response to a self antigen is 'inappropriate'. The hypersensitivity reactions were classified by Gell and Coombs, according to the speed of the reaction and the immune mechanisms involved. Although they are classified separately, in practice they do not necessarily occur in isolation

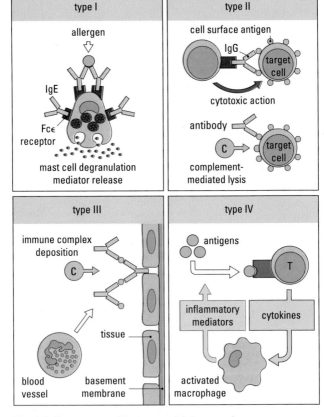

Fig. 4.8 Four types of hypersensitivity reaction.

from each other. Moreover, several different immune reactions may be subsumed in a single type.

Type I (Immediate) hypersensitivity is seen in allergic asthma, hayfever and some types of eczema. It develops within minutes of exposure to antigen, and is dependent on the activation of mast cells and the release of mediators of acute inflammation. Mast cells bind IgE via their surface Fcε receptors, and when antigen crosslinks the IgE, the mast cells degranulate, releasing vasoactive amines which produce acute inflammation. Prostaglandins and leukotrienes, produced by arachidonic acid metabolism, contribute to a delayed component of the reaction which often develops hours after the original exposure to antigen.

Type II (Antibody-mediated) hypersensitivity is caused by antibody to cell surface antigens and components of the extracellular matrix. These antibodies can sensitize the cells for antibody-dependent cytotoxic attack by K cells or for complement-mediated lysis. Type II hypersensitivity is seen in the destruction of red cells in transfusion reactions and in haemolytic disease of the newborn. Tissue destruction in autoimmune diseases such as myasthenia gravis, Goodpasture's syndrome and pemphigus is primarily antibody-mediated.

Type III (Immune-complex-mediated) hypersensitivity is caused by the deposition of antigen/antibody complexes in tissue and blood vessels. This tends to occur at sites of filtration such as the glomerulus. The complexes activate complement and attract polymorphs and macrophages to the site. These cells may exocytose their granule contents and release reactive oxygen and nitrogen intermediates to cause local tissue damage. The antigens in the complexes may come from persistent pathogenic infections (eg. malaria), from inhaled antigens (eg. extrinsic allergic alveolitis) or from the host's own tissue (in autoimmune disease). These conditions are all characterized by a high antigen load, which may be associated with a weak or ineffective antibody response.

Type IV (Delayed) hypersensitivity arises more than 24 hours after encounter with the antigen and is mediated by antigen-sensitized CD4+ T cells, which release cytokines, attracting macrophages to the site and activating them. The macrophages produce tissue damage which may develop into chronic granulomatous reactions if the antigen persists. This type of hypersensitivity is seen in skin contact reactions and in the response to some chronic pathogens, such as *Mycobacterium leprae*, *M. tuberculosis* and *Schistosoma* spp.

TYPE I (IMMEDIATE) HYPERSENSITIVITY

Allergy, originally meaning altered reactivity on a second contact with an antigen, now means type I hypersensitivity. These reactions are mediated by IgE, and indicate a TH2-type response.

Sensitization in this context is the process by which a susceptible individual develops an allergen-specific IgE response. Typical allergens are pollens and house-dust-mite faeces. The IgE may bind to the high-affinity FcεR on mast cells, thereby sensitizing them for triggering by the allergen.

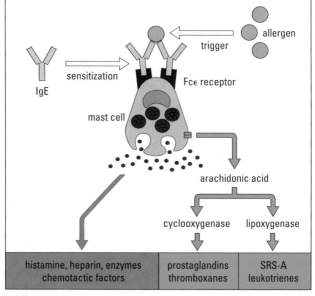

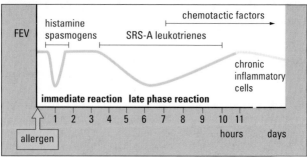

Fig. 4.9 Type I hypersensitivity.

Triggering of mast cells occurs when antigen crosslinks the cell surface IgE, causing an influx of Ca^{++}, resulting in degranulation and activation of phospholipase A2. Mast cells can also be directly triggered by anaphylatoxins, C3a and C5a.

Phospholipase A2 is a membrane-associated enzyme which releases arachidonic acid, the initial substrate for the lipoxygenase pathway, which produces leukotrienes, and the cyclooxygenase pathway, which produces prostaglandins and thromboxanes.

Atopy describes conditions which manifest type I hypersensitivity, including asthma, hayfever and eczema. They tend to cluster in families. These reactions are exemplified opposite by allergic asthma induced by breathing an allergen.

Immediate and Late-phase reactions. Following bronchial provocation with an allergen, there is an immediate reduction in airway patency, measured as a fall in forced expiratory volume (FEV), caused by histamine, prostaglandins, and kinins, and via the action of PAF on platelets. After several hours a late-phase reaction develops caused primarily by leukotrienes and cytokines. Inflammatory cells, including macrophages, basophils and other polymorphs, arrive under chemotactic influences. Eosinophil granule proteins are highly toxic for airway epithelium. Analogous immediate and late reactions occur in allergic skin reactions.

SRS-A (Slow Reacting Substance-A), a mediator of the late-phase reaction, consists primarily of leukotrienes C4 and D4. LTC4 is a particularly powerful bronchoconstrictor.

Anaphylaxis is a systemic type I reaction seen in sensitized animals injected with allergen. The release of vasoactive amines and spasmogens causes smooth muscle contraction, increased vascular permeability and a fall in blood pressure. Respiratory or circulatory failure may ensue. Anaphylactic reactions may occur in man, for example caused by bee venom in a sensitive individual.

Passive Cutaneous Anaphylaxis (PCA) is an assay for antigen-specific IgE in which an animal is sensitized by subcutaneous injection of test serum and then challenged with allergen. If specific IgE is present in the serum, the local mast cells degranulate, causing increased local vascular permeability.

Prick test is used to determine an individual's (type I) sensitivity to allergens, which are pricked onto the skin. Sensitive individuals generate a wheal-and-flare reaction.

TYPE II (ANTIBODY-MEDIATED) HYPERSENSITIVITY

Type II hypersensitivity is caused by antibody directed to membranes and cell surface antigens. Complement may be activated, and effector cells with Fcγ receptors and C3 receptors can then engage the target tissue. Membrane attack complexes may also be formed, to potentiate the damage. The site of damage depends on the antibodies involved.

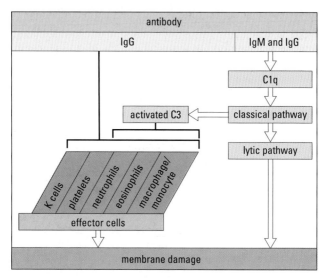

Fig. 4.10 Type II hypersensitivity.

Transfusion reactions occur when mismatched donor blood is infused into a recipient. The recipient may have naturally occurring antibodies to the foreign cells, as happens with the ABO blood group system, or they may develop after infusion. The antibodies can cause complement-dependent lysis or sequestration of the sensitized cells in spleen and liver.

Blood groups are systems of allotypically variable erythrocyte surface antigens, some of which occur on other tissues also. The more common ones are listed in Figure 4.11.

Haemolytic Disease of the Newborn (HDNB) is caused by maternal antibodies to foetal red cells, which cross the placenta and destroy them. The mother becomes sensitized by foetal red cells entering her circulation at birth, so that the first child is usually unaffected. The most common cases involve Rhesus-negative mothers carrying Rhesus-positive children.

Rhesus prophylaxis is the administration of anti-Rhesus D antibody to Rhesus-negative mothers immediately after they have delivered a Rhesus-positive child, in order to destroy the Rh+ cells and thus, prevent them sensitizing the mother.

Autoimmune haemolytic anaemia is caused by autoantibodies to red cells, producing cell destruction by lysis or sequestration. The antibodies may be either 'warm agglutinins' or 'cold agglutinins' depending on the temperature at which they bind.

Myasthenia Gravis (MG) is a disease with muscle weakness, owing to impaired neuromuscular transmission, partly caused by autoantibodies to acetylcholine receptors.

Pemphigus is an autoimmune disease in which antibodies are directed against desmosomes between keratinocytes. This produces detachment of the epidermis and blistering.

Goodpasture's syndrome has a type II reaction in which autoantibodies damage lung and kidney basement membranes.

system	gene loci	antigens	phenotype frequencies	
ABO	1	A, B or 0	A B AB 0	42% 8% 3% 47%
Rhesus	3 closely linked loci: major antigen=RhD	C or c D or d E or e	RhD$^+$ RhD$^-$	85% 15%
Kell	1	K or k	K k	9% 91%
Duffy	1	Fy^a, Fy^b or Fy	Fy^{a}Fy^b Fy^a Fy^b Fy	46% 20% 34% 0.1%
MN	1	M or N	MM MN NN	28% 50% 22%

Fig. 4.11 Five major human blood group systems.

TYPE III (IMMUNE-COMPLEX-MEDIATED) HYPERSENSITIVITY

Immune complexes are combinations of antigen and antibody, often with associated complement components.

Immune complex deposition. Type III hypersensitivity results from the deposition of immune complexes in blood vessel walls and tissues. Complexes can activate platelets (in man) and basophils via Fc receptors, to release vasoactive amines which cause endothelial cell retraction and increased vascular permeability, leading to complex deposition. Complexes also activate complement, releasing C3a and C5a, both of which activate basophils, while C5a is chemotactic for neutrophils. Phagocytes which are unable to endocytose the deposited complexes, release granule contents and ROIs, causing local tissue damage. Complexes tend to deposit at sites of high pressure, filtration or turbulence, particularly the kidney.

Immune complex clearance. In man, circulating complexes are normally taken up by erythrocytes and carried to the liver, where they are transferred to, and degraded by, phagocytes. Factors

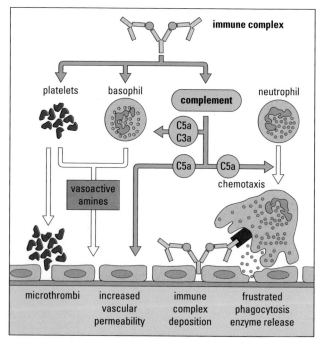

Fig. 4.12 Immune complex deposition.

which affect clearance include: 1) Size of the complexes; 2) Class and affinity of the antibody; 3) Valency of the antigen; 4) The amount of complex. This last factor explains why immune complex disease occurs in infections which release large amounts of antigen, and in autoimmune diseases where there is a ready supply of autoantigen.

Immune complex diseases result when excessive immune complex deposition occurs in particular organs (see Fig 4.13).

Serum sickness is a type III reaction which occurs in individuals injected with foreign serum. Antibodies are made to the serum antigens and there is massive immune complex formation, producing arthritis and nephritis.

Arthus reaction is a skin reaction seen as an area of redness and swelling which is maximal 5–6 hours after intradermal injection of antigen. It is caused by IgG binding to the injected antigen and triggering inflammation by type III mechanisms.

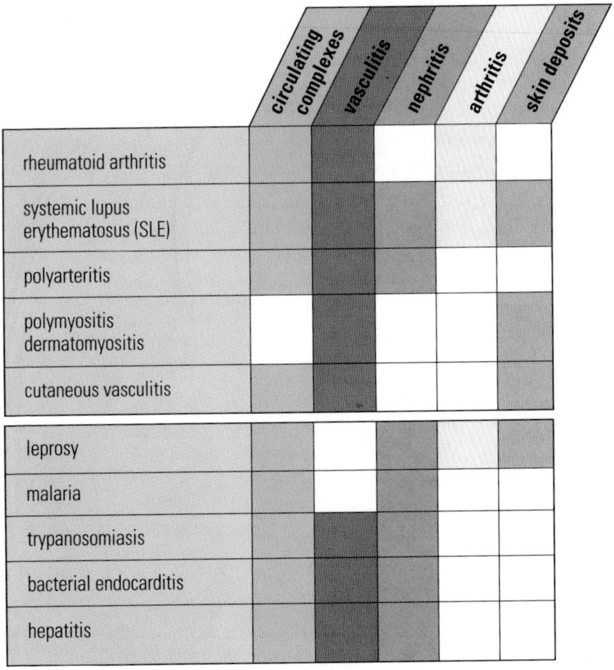

	circulating complexes	vasculitis	nephritis	arthritis	skin deposits
rheumatoid arthritis					
systemic lupus erythematosus (SLE)					
polyarteritis					
polymyositis dermatomyositis					
cutaneous vasculitis					
leprosy					
malaria					
trypanosomiasis					
bacterial endocarditis					
hepatitis					

Fig. 4.13 Immune complex diseases: sites of deposition.

TYPE IV (DELAYED) HYPERSENSITIVITY (DTH)

This includes a number of reactions which are maximal at more than 12 hours after challenge with antigen, and which are dependent on antigen-reactive T cells, rather than antibody. The cells responsible are a functionally defined subgroup of CD4+ TH cells, previously referred to as TD cells. At least four types of reaction have been described, but they may occur concomitantly or sequentially in the reaction to a particular antigen. For example, if an antigenic stimulus persists, a tuberculin-type reaction may develop into a granuloma.

Jones Mote reactions (Cutaneous basophil hypersensitivity) appear within 24 hours of skin challenge with antigen. The area beneath the epidermis becomes infiltrated with basophils over 1–6 days, with maximal skin swelling on day 1.

Contact hypersensitivity produces an eczematous skin reaction in sensitized humans, which is maximal 48 hours after contact with the allergen. The allergens may be large molecules or small haptens (eg. nickel) which attach to normal body proteins and modify them. Langerhans' cells pick up these antigens and present them to T cells in local lymph nodes. On rechallenge with the allergen, sensitized T cells migrate into the skin site, producing a reaction characterized by mononuclear cell infiltration, with oedema and microvesicle formation in the epidermis. The dermis is usually infiltrated by an increased number of leucocytes.

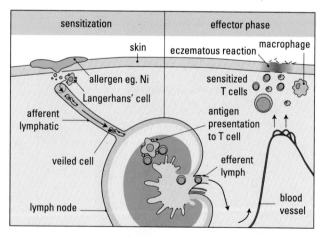

Fig. 4.14 Sensitization and effector phases of contact hypersensitivity.

Tuberculin-type hypersensitivity was originally a reaction produced by subcutaneous injection of tuberculin in patients with tuberculosis, who responded with fever and swelling at the injection site. The term usually refers to the skin reaction induced by antigen which is maximal at 48 hours after challenge and consists of lymphocytes and mononuclear phagocytes. If the antigenic stimulus persists, a granulomatous reaction may develop. This type of reaction may be induced in a sensitized subject by several microbial and non-microbial antigens.

Granulomatous reactions develop where there is a persistent stimulus which macrophages cannot eliminate. Non-antigenic particles (eg. talc) induce non-immunological granulomas, while persistent pathogens such as *Mycobacterium* spp. and *Schistosomula* spp. induce immunological granulomas. The lesion consists of a palisade of epithelioid cells and macrophages surrounding the infectious agent, which is in turn surrounded by a cuff of lymphocytes. Collagenous capsules may also develop around some pathogens because of fibroblast proliferation.

Epithelioid cells, large flattened cells with large amounts of endoplasmic reticulum, are seen in granulomas and are thought to be derived from macrophages, although they have fewer phagosomes than macrophages. Nevertheless, cytokine formation by these cells (eg. TNF) is important in the granulomatous reaction.

Giant cells are large multinucleated cells present in granulomas, which are derived from the fusion of macrophages and/or epithelioid cells.

TH1-type responses. Some diseases (eg. multiple sclerosis) appear to centre around overactive cell-mediated immune reponses. Such TH1 reactions are particularly damaging in the CNS. This is not type IV hypersensitivity as originally defined, since an inducing antigen has not been identified, but some similarities are present.

Migration Inhibition Test (MIT). This assay detects sensitized T cells. Test cells are packed with monocytes and antigen in capillary tubes and then cultured on agar plates. If antigen-sensitive T cells are present, they release cytokines (MIF, IL-8 etc.) which limit the migration of the monocytes.

Patch test is used to assess type IV contact hypersensitivity to allergens. The allergen is applied to the skin and the development of an eczematous reaction 48 hours later indicates that the subject is sensitive to that allergen.

Immunological Techniques

5

ASSAYS FOR ANTIGEN AND ANTIBODY

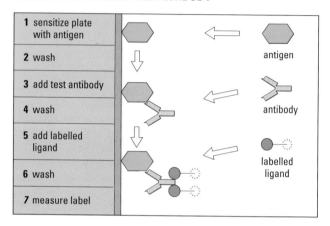

1 sensitize plate with antigen	
2 wash	antigen
3 add test antibody	
4 wash	antibody
5 add labelled ligand	
6 wash	labelled ligand
7 measure label	

Fig. 5.1 Radioimmunoassay.

Radioimmunoassay (RIA) includes a variety of techniques which use radiolabelled reagents to detect antigen or antibody. Antibody may be detected using plates sensitized with antigen (Fig. 5.1). Test antibody is applied and this is detected by the addition of a radiolabelled ligand specific for that antibody. The amount of ligand bound to the plate is proportional to the amount of test antibody. RIA ligands are usually antibody molecules or protein A, covalently bound to ^{125}I.

Protein A and Protein G are cell wall components of staphylococci, which bind specifically to IgG (Fc) of most species at a site between $C\gamma2$ and $C\gamma3$. Protein G binds a wider range of Igs than protein A.

Streptavidin/biotin reagents are used in many immunoassays (eg. RIA and ELISA) to amplify detection and reduce background. Streptavidin binds biotin with very high affinity. For example, the antibody in Fig. 5.3 (ELISA) could be biotinylated and this would then be detected with enzyme coupled to streptavidin.

Radioallergosorbent Test (RAST) is a specialized RIA to detect antigen-specific IgE. Antigen is covalently coupled to cellulose discs, and specific IgE is detected using radiolabelled anti-IgE.

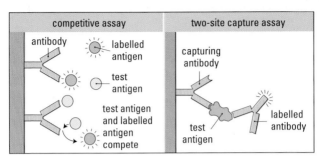

Fig. 5.2 Competition and sandwich (capture) radioimmunoassays.

Competition radioimmunoassay is the classical RIA. It is used to detect antigens. Specific antibody is bound to a solid phase, and a mixture of test (unlabelled) and labelled antigen is applied. Labelled and unlabelled antigens compete with each other for the antibodies' binding sites. The greater the amount of test antigen that is present, the less labelled antigen will bind to the antibody. Calibration curves using known quantities of unlabelled antigen are established. The technique is often used for assaying hormones.

Radioimmunosorbent Test (RIST) is a competition RIA used to detect IgE (the antigen in this assay), in which test IgE is competed with labelled IgE on plates sensitized with anti-IgE.

Sandwich (capture) immunoassays use antibody bound to the solid-phase to capture molecules (antigens) from the test solution, which are then detected with a second labelled antibody. For example, solid phase anti-IFN-γ captures IFN-γ from the test solution, and this is detected with a second labelled antibody which binds a different site on the IFN-γ. Such assays can detect antigens at around 1 ng/ml and are often used to detect (eg.) cytokines.

Immunoradiometric Assay (IRMA) is a test for antigen in which excess specific labelled antibody is added to the test antigen which binds and neutralizes some of the antibody – free antibody is removed by adding solid-phase antigen. The labelled antibody still in solution remains bound to the test antigen, so the radioactivity of the solution is proportional to the amount of test antigen.

Farr assay uses radiolabelled antigens to detect specific antibody. The test antibody is first mixed with the labelled antigen, then the antibodies are precipitated using a specific precipitating reagent, eg. solid-phase protein A. The amount of precipitated antigen is proportional to the amount of specific antibody.

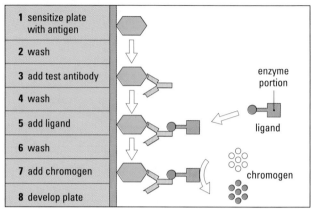

| 1 sensitize plate with antigen |
| 2 wash |
| 3 add test antibody |
| 4 wash |
| 5 add ligand |
| 6 wash |
| 7 add chromogen |
| 8 develop plate |

enzyme portion

ligand

chromogen

Fig. 5.3 Enzyme-linked immunosorbent assay (ELISA).

Enzyme-Linked Immunosorbent Assay (ELISA) is used for detecting antibodies or antigens in ways analogous to RIAs, but with the substitution of an enzyme for the radioactive isotope; eg. antigen is absorbed to a solid phase and test antibody is added, which is detected using enzyme-labelled protein G (binds IgG). Enzymes such as peroxidase and phosphatase are often used. In the final stage, a chromogenic substrate is added, which generates a coloured end-product in the presence of the enzyme portion of the ligand. The optical density of this solution is measured after a defined period. This is proportional to the amount of the enzyme, which in turn is related to the amount of test antibody. By comparison with RIA, this test has the advantage of stable reagents, but is usually less sensitive and less linear.

Homogenous Enzyme Immunoassays (EMITs) are a group of assays to detect antigen using the antigen coupled to an enzyme in such a way that the activity of the enzyme is altered when the antigen binds to the antibody.

Nephelometry is an assay used to detect antigen or antibody by the formation of immune complexes. The complexes make the solution turbid and this can be detected by light scatter.

Fluorescence Immunoassay (FIA) is analogous to RIAs, but substitutes fluoresceinated reagents for the radiolabelled material. The method has the advantage that fluorescent reagents may be detected instantaneously, but problems can arise with the intrinsic fluorescence of the test material and also with the availability of suitable reagents. Some fluorescent reagents respond differently when they are bound to antibody than when free. In this case it is not necessary to separate bound and free fractions of the fluorescent reagent. For example:

Fluorescence quenching is the reduction of fluorescence emitted by an antibody (or antigen) when it forms a complex. For example, this occurs when a hapten, which absorbs radiation at 350nm, binds to an antibody. Normally, antibody illuminated at 280nm fluoresces at 350nm, but if the hapten is bound at the binding site some of the fluorescence is absorbed (quenched).

Fluorescence enhancement is the increased fluorescence produced by some haptens when bound to antibody. The energy is absorbed from the antibody and emitted with the wavelength characteristic of the hapten.

Fluorescence polarization. If polarized light is directed at a fluorescent molecule it is absorbed and emitted shortly afterwards, during which time the molecules move at random so that the fluorescent emission shows reduced polarization. If, however, the fluorescent molecule is bound to an antibody it has less rotational freedom and the initial polarization is retained in the emission.

Fluorescence (resonance) energy transfer is used to determine the proximity of two molecules on a cell surface. One is labelled with a fluoresceinated antibody (donor) and the other with a rhodaminated antibody (acceptor). The cells are illuminated at the donor's wavelength. If the two molecules are sufficiently close (<10nm), energy is transferred between the fluorochromes and is detected as an emission at the acceptor's wavelength (red).

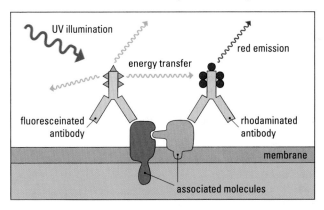

Fig. 5.4 Resonance energy transfer.

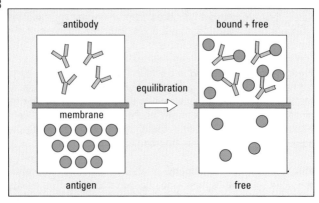

Fig. 5.5 Equilibrium dialysis.

Equilibrium dialysis is a method for determining antibody affinity, in which a dialysable antigen and the test antibody are placed in chambers on opposite sides of a membrane. The system is left until the concentration of free antigen is the same on either side of the membrane (equilibrium), and then the solutions are sampled. The average affinity (K_0) is defined as the reciprocal of the free antigen concentration when half of the antibody's combining sites are occupied; for IgG with two sites: Affinity, $K_0 = 1/[Ag_{free}]$.

Chaotropic dissociation assay is used to measure the heterogeneity of antibody affinities in, for example, serum. Immune complexes are dissociated in buffers of varying strengths at high or low pH or in chaotropic reagents. Low-affinity antibodies dissociate in lower strength reagents.

Haemagglutination. This term covers a number of techniques for detecting antibodies, based on the agglutination of red blood cells. The antigen may either be a red cell antigen, or the antigen (sensitizing antigen) required can be chemically linked to the cell surface. For the test, the antibody is titrated in wells and the red cells added. If antibody to the red cell is present, the cells are agglutinated and sink as a mat to the bottom of the well, but if it is absent, they roll down the sloping sides of the well to form a pellet.

Direct and Indirect Coombs' tests are haemagglutination assays which detect antibodies to red cell antigens. The direct Coombs' test identifies antibodies which can themselves crosslink the red cells. The indirect Coombs' test detects antibodies which cannot crosslink the cells alone (eg. because there are too few antigens). Agglutination is achieved by adding a second-layer anti-antibody.

Complement fixation test detects antibody (or antigen). Test antibody is mixed with the antigen and a small amount of active complement. If antibody is present, complexes form and fix the complement, but if none is present, active complement remains. Active complement is detected (if complexes did not form) by adding antibody-sensitized red cells (EA), which lyse if complement is present. (To detect antigen, specific antibody is mixed with the test solution and complement.)

Immunoblotting (Western blotting) is used to identify proteins which have been separated by gel electrophoresis and then transferred to a membrane (blot). The blot is incubated with radiolabelled or enzyme-labelled antibody which binds to antigens on the blot. The bound antibody can be detected by using a secondlayer radiolabelled anti-antibody, or enzyme-conjugated antibody (cf. RAI and ELISA).

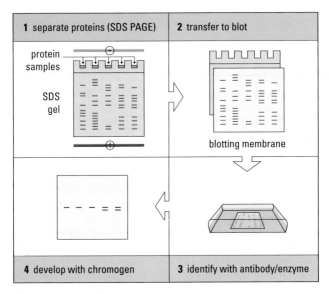

Fig. 5.6 Immunoblotting.

Immunoprecipitation is used for characterizing the antigen recognized by a monoclonal antibody, particularly where the antigen is denatured by immunoblotting. The antigen mixture is labelled (radiolabel, biotinylation etc.) and precipitated in solution with the monoclonal antibody and coprecipitating agent (protein A, anti-Ig antibody etc.). The precipitate is then separated on SDS PAGE and the labelled antigen localized.

Precipitin reactions. When antigen and antibody react together near their equivalence point, they often form crosslinked precipitates. If the reaction occurs in a supporting medium, such as an agar gel, the reactants form precipitin arcs, which can be used to identify antigens and antibodies in complex mixtures.

Immunodouble diffusion (Ouchterlony) is used to distinguish antigens in mixtures. The reactants are placed in holes punched in the gel, and diffuse together. The precipitin arcs may show one of three patterns. Where two arcs are fused, this indicates identity between the antigens. If they form independently, the antigens are not identical, and if the arcs are fused but with a spur, then the antigens are partially identical, but one antigen contains epitopes which the other lacks.

Countercurrent electrophoresis is a technique for detecting antigens or antibodies by forcing them to move together in an electric field. The technique is related to, but more sensitive than, immunodouble diffusion.

Single Radial Immunodiffusion (SRID) (Mancini) is used to quantitate antibody. Test antibody is put in wells in an antigen-containing gel, and diffuses out to form precipitin rings when it reaches equivalence. The area of the ring is proportional to antibody concentration. Antigen can be measured similarly using antibody-containing gels.

Rocket electrophoresis is a modification of SRID in which antigens are quantitated by electrophoresing them through an antibody-containing gel, the pH of which is selected so that the antibodies are neutrally charged and immobile. The antigen moves towards the anode, forming a rocket-shaped precipitin arc, where the height of the rocket is proportional to antigen concentrations.

Immunoelectrophoresis (IEP) is a technique in which mixtures of antigen are first separated in an electric field according to their charge, and are then precipitated with antiserum from a trough lying parallel to the separated antigens.

Crossed electrophoresis (Laurell) first separates antigens according to their charge in an electric field, in the first dimension. Then the antigens are electrophoresed into an antibody-containing gel at right angles to the first separation. The area under the precipitin arcs is proportional to antigen concentration. This technique is useful for quantitating the different forms of an antigen, for example C3 and C3c, which share epitopes but have different charges.

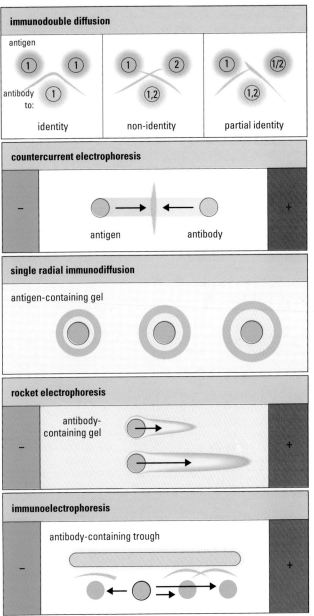

Fig. 5.7 Agar gel immunoprecipitation techniques for antigens and antibody.

Immunoabsorption is used specifically to remove particular anti-bodies from a solution, by the addition of a solid-phase antigen immunoabsorbent. Immunoabsorbents – ie. solid-phase antigens or antibodies – include cells, chemically crosslinked antigen precipitates and proteins coupled to solid supports.

Affinity chromatography is used to isolate pure antibodies. A column is prepared from antigen covalently coupled to an inert solid phase such as crosslinked dextran beads. The antibody-containing solution is run into the column in neutral buffer. Specific antibody binds to the antigen, while unbound antibody and other proteins are washed through. The specific antibody is eluted using a buffer which dissociates the antigen/antibody bond, that is, high or low pH or denaturing agents. By using antibody bound to the solid phase the technique can be used to isolate antigen.

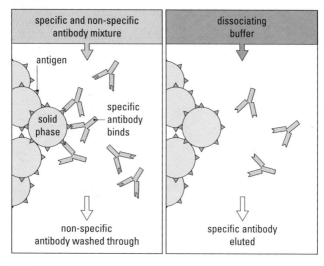

Fig. 5.8 Affinity chromatography.

Immunofluorescence is a general method for identifying anti-gens in tissue sections and on cells, or for identifying antibodies to them, as follows:

Direct immunofluoresence. The antibody is covalently coupled to a fluorescent molecule, such as fluorescein, rhodamine or Texas red, which is then incubated with the cells or a frozen tissue sec-tion. (Some antibodies bind to wax-embedded sections, but not all.) The antibody binds to the antigen and this is then visualized by observing the material under a microscope with incident UV light.

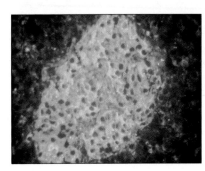

**Fig. 5.9
Immunofluorescence:
islet cell autoanti-
bodies.** Courtesy of
Dr B. Dean.

Indirect immunofluorescence. In this technique the section is incubated with the test antibody, which is then visualized by the addition of a second-layer fluorescent anti-antibody. The amplification produced by the second antibody increases the sensitivity of the assay, and by using class- or subclass-specific reagents particular isotypes can be identified in the test antibody. This technique is of particular value for identifying antibodies to tissue antigens, as illustrated above, where antibodies to a pancreatic islet of Langerhans in diabetic serum were identified by indirect immunofluorescence using a frozen section of pancreas.

Immunohistochemistry is similar to immunofluorescence, but enzyme-labelled conjugates and chromogens are substituted for the fluorescent conjugates. Sections are viewed by light microscopy.

Capping occurs when antibodies bind and crosslink the surface antigens on a live cell. The antigens aggregate at one pole of the cell, appearing as a (fluorescent) cap. The cap is then internalized (capped off). Treatment of cells with metabolic inhibitors (eg. azide) prevents capping. Co-capping is used to determine whether two different cell surface antigens are independent, in which case they form separate caps, with specific antibodies, or associated, when they form a single cap (co-cap).

Photobleaching recovery is used to measure the lateral mobility of molecules on a cell membrane. A molecule is labelled by a fluorescent antibody and a spot of the membrane is bleached by extended illumination with UV light. The rate at which unbleached labelled molecules re-enter the bleached area after the UV is shut off is a measure of the rate of molecular mobility.

Immunogold labelling is used to identify antigens in electron microscopy, using antibodies coupled to tiny gold particles.

ISOLATION OF CELLS

Ficoll gradients are used to isolate cells of different densities. In particular they are used in the purification of lymphocytes. A diluted blood sample is layered onto the Ficoll and centrifuged. Since red blood cells and polymorphs are denser than Ficoll they sediment to the bottom, whilst the lymphocytes and some macrophages remain at the interface. Lymphocyte populations may be further depleted of macrophages by adherence, or by letting the phagocytes take up iron filings and then removing them with a magnet.

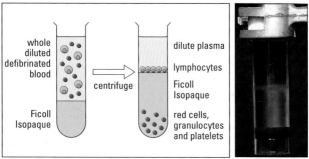

Fig. 5.10 Separation of lymphocytes on a Ficoll Isopaque gradient.

Adherence. Macrophages have the property of adhering to plastic; they may be removed from the cell suspensions by plating on plastic dishes to which they adhere.

Panning uses plastic plates sensitized with antigen or antibody (cf. RIA). Mixtures of cells are incubated on the plate, and cells with receptors for the sensitizing agent bind to it. For example, cells with an antigen receptor will bind to an antigen-coated plate. The technique is often used to deplete cells of a specific sub-population, but the bound cells can sometimes be recovered by chilling or digesting the plate with enzyme.

Antibody/Complement depletion. Specific cell populations can be removed from a mixture by lysis with antibody and complement.

Immunomagnetic beads are an efficient way of isolating cell populations in bulk. The cells are mixed with magnetic beads coupled to a particular antibody (eg. anti-CD4); they may then be rapidly removed or isolated by placing the tube in a magnetic field.

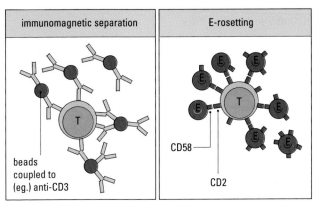

| immunomagnetic separation | E-rosetting |

Fig. 5.11 T cell separation by rosetting or immunomagnetic beads.

Rosetting is a method of isolating cells by allowing them to associate with red blood cells. Lymphocytes become surrounded (rosette) with the red cells and may then be isolated by sedimentation through Ficoll gradients. Human T cells have receptors for sheep erythrocytes (E) and so may be isolated by mixing with the sheep cells and separating the rosettes produced (Fig. 5.11). Cells which have Fc receptors for IgM or IgG can be isolated by mixing with red cells sensitized with antibody of the appropriate class. The antibody crosslinks the red cell to the Fc receptor and the rosettes are then isolated.

Antigen suicide is used to deplete those cells of a population which bind a particular antigen, by supplying them with highly radioactive antigen. This is taken up and kills the cell. A modification of this technique, to kill proliferating cells, is to add bromodeoxyuridine, which they incorporate. Illumination with UV light activates this metabolite to kill the cells.

Flow cytometry is a technique that measures the characteristics of individual cells, including size, granularity and fluorescence, as they pass through a flow cytometer in a stream of droplets. Cells may be stained with up to three different fluorescent antibodies to quantitate the surface density of three different molecules. Different populations of cells are then identified according to the expression of these molecules.

Fluorescence-Activated Cell Sorter (FACS) is a machine which carries out flow cytometry on a population of cells and can then sort the cells into different subpopulations. The parameters for the sort (size, fluorescence intensity etc.) are set by the operator.

CLONES AND CELL LINES

A clone is a group of cells derived from a single original cell; they are therefore genetically identical. A cell line is a group of cells grown in defined conditions from an initially heterogenous population. Only occasionally will such a line be monoclonal.

Hybridomas are cells produced by the physical fusion of two different cells. Polyethylene glycol (PEG) and Sendai virus are often used to effect the fusion. A hybridoma cell and its progeny contain some chromosomes from each fusion partner, although some others are usually lost.

Monoclonal antibodies are homogenous antibodies produced by a single clone. They are usually made from hybridomas, which are prepared by fusing immunized mouse or rat spleen cells with a non-secretor myeloma using PEG. The fusion mixture is plated out in HAT medium: HAT contains Hypoxanthine, Aminopterin and Thymidine. Aminopterin blocks a metabolic pathway which can be bypassed if hypoxanthine and thymidine are present, but the myeloma cells lack this bypass and consequently die in HAT medium. Spleen cells also die naturally in culture after 1–2 weeks, but fused cells survive since they have the immortality of the myeloma and the metabolic bypass of the spleen cells. Some of the fused cells secrete antibody, and supernatants are tested in a specific assay. Wells which produce the desired antibody are then cloned. Human B cells can be immortalized by transformation with Epstein-Barr virus. By comparison with polyclonal antisera, monoclonal antibodies are well defined, but not necessarily more specific or of higher affinity.

Cloning is a process in which a cell population is diluted successively and set up in culture so that there are wells containing only one cell. The progeny of this cell are grown on as a clone. Alternatively, the cultures may be grown in soft agar to prevent them spreading, and colonies are isolated by micromanipulation.

Phage display antibodies. An alternative way of producing monoclonal antibodies or antibody fragments is by using molecular biological techniques. Mixed mRNA for antibody V_H and V_L domains are amplified and crosslinked with a spacer to give a gene for an antibody Fv fragment (contains one antigen-binding site). The synthetic gene is inserted into a vector (phage), which expresses the Fv on its tips. The phage are selected according to their ability to bind to antigen-coated plates, and positive phage are used to transfect bacteria, which now synthesize the required Fv fragments.

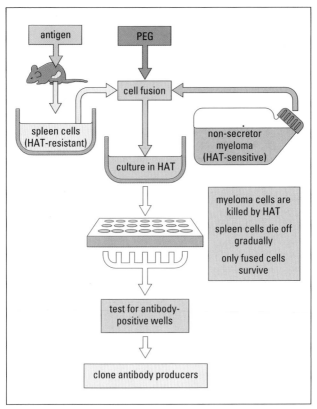

Fig. 5.12 Monoclonal antibody production.

T cell lines are produced by culturing a population of primed T cells in the presence of antigen and interleukin-2. The antigen must be presented to the T cells by APCs, usually macrophages or thymocytes, which have been treated to block their metabolism. T cell activity is assayed by antigen-specific proliferation.

Proliferation is usually measured by the uptake of radiolabelled metabolites required for DNA or RNA synthesis, such as ^{125}I-uridine deoxyribose or ^{3}H-thymidine. The uptake of these metabolites is measured by harvesting the cells and counting the incorporated radioactivity.

Cell harvester is a machine which semi-automatically aspirates cell cultures, deposits them onto small paper filters and washes away free radioactive metabolites.

CELLULAR FUNCTIONS

Plaque-Forming Cells (PFCs) are antibody-secreting cells measured in an assay where each secreting cell produces a clear zone of lysis (plaque) in a layer of antigen-sensitized red blood cells (Fig. 5.13).

Direct and Indirect plaques. Indirect plaques measure antigen-specific IgG producers. The test lymphocytes are mixed and incubated with antigen-sensitized red cells (cf. haemagglutination). Antibody from specific B cells binds to the antigen on the red cells, and the addition of antibody to IgG together with complement causes complement fixation on the red cells, producing a plaque of lysed cells. Direct plaques measure the numbers of antigen-specific IgM-producing cells. IgM is capable of fixing complement without the addition of a second-layer antibody. Thus IgG- and IgM-producing cells can be quantitated separately. Total antibody-producing cells (not just the antigen-specific ones) are measured by the reverse plaque assay in which the red cells are sensitized with anti-Ig or protein A.

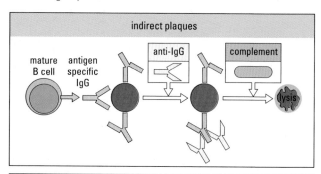

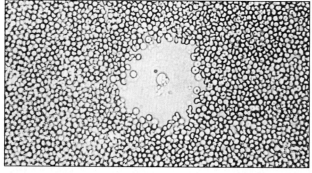

Fig. 5.13 Plaque-forming cell assay (top) and plaque (bottom).

Elispot assays are enzyme immunoassays used to quantitate antigen-specific cells, which are analogous to the PFC technique. Antibody-forming cells are detected by overlaying lymphocytes in agar on a plate sensitized with the specific antigen. Specific antibody binds to the antigen around the cells secreting it. This can then be detected by enzyme immunoassay, producing a coloured spot around the active cells. The technique is also used to detect the numbers of cells secreting a particular cytokine. For example, active T_H1 cells can be detected by overlaying them on plates sensitized with antibody to IFN-γ to capture the IFN-γ. The spot of cytokine is detected using another antibody to a different epitope of the IFN-γ.

In-situ hybridization is a useful molecular biological technique to detect expression of particular proteins in tissues (eg. cytokines). Tissue sections are hybridized with radiolabelled cDNA of the protein in question, and the cellular localization of mRNA for that protein determined by autoradiography.

Chromium release (cytotoxicity) assay is used to measure the activity of cytotoxic cells. The target cells are first mixed with radioactive ^{51}Cr, which is taken up by viable cells. These are then incubated with the test leucocytes. If the test cells damage the targets, the ^{51}Cr is released and can be measured in the supernatant.

NBT (Nitroblue Tetrazolium) reduction is a standard test for the oxidative burst in neutrophils.

Adhesion assays are used to detect interactions between different cell populations, particularly leucocytes and endothelium. The simplest method is to examine the coculture of leucocytes and endothelium *in vitro* under the microscope and count the numbers of bound cells on top of the endothelium (and therefore phase-bright) and the migrated cells beneath the endothelium (phase-dark). To quantitate the bound and migrated populations more systematically, the applied leucocytes are prelabelled with ^{51}Cr. After being washed to remove unbound cells, the coculture is lysed, releasing the ^{51}Cr, which is a measure of the proportion of bound + migrated leucocytes. Adhesion *in situ* is measured by the Stamper-Woodruff assay, in which leucocytes are overlaid on frozen tissue sections containing the blood vessels under investigation. Sections are examined under the microscope for evidence of leucocyte adhesion to the vessels. This technique was first used to identify the function of high endothelial cells (HEVs) in lymph nodes. The molecules involved in adhesion have been identified both *in vitro* and *in situ* by adhesion-blocking with specific antibodies (eg. anti-LFA-1).